WHEN LONGING BECOMES YOUR LOVER

Breaking from Infatuation, Rejection,
and Perfectionism to Find Authentic Love:
A True Story of Overcoming Limerence

AMANDA McCRACKEN

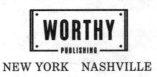

WORTHY
PUBLISHING

NEW YORK   NASHVILLE

Worthy Books
Hachette Book Group
1290 Avenue of the Americas
New York, NY 10104
worthypublishing.com
@WorthyPub

First Edition: February 2026

Worthy is a division of Hachette Book Group, Inc. The Worthy Books name and logo are registered trademarks of Hachette Book Group, Inc.

The publisher is not responsible for websites (or their content) that are not owned by the publisher.

The Hachette Speakers Bureau provides a wide range of authors for speaking events. To find out more, visit hachettespeakersbureau.com or email HachetteSpeakers@hbgusa.com.

Worthy Books may be purchased in bulk for business, educational, or promotional use. For information, please contact your local bookseller or email the Hachette Book Group Special Markets Department at Special.Markets@hbgusa.com.

Print book interior design by Sheryl Kober

Library of Congress Cataloging-in-Publication Data

Name: McCracken, Amanda author
Title: When longing becomes your lover: breaking from infatuation, rejection, and perfectionism to find authentic love: a true story of overcoming limerence / Amanda McCracken.
Description: First edition. | New York: Worthy Books, 2026. | Includes bibliographical references.
Identifiers: LCCN 2025038691 | ISBN 9781546008538 hardcover | ISBN 9781546008545 trade paperback | ISBN 9781546008552 ebook
Subjects: LCSH: McCracken, Amanda | Journalists—United States—Biography | Women journalists—United States—Biography | Infatuation—United States | LCGFT: Autobiographies
Classification: LCC PN4874.M3635 A3 2026
LC record available at https://lccn.loc.gov/2025038691

ISBNs: 9781546008538 (hardcover); 9781546008552 (ebook)

Printed in Canada

MRQ-T

10 9 8 7 6 5 4 3 2 1

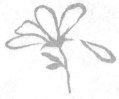

To Dave for trusting me
To Moorea for inspiring me
To Patrice and Mike for believing in me
To Thom for modeling resilience

CONTENTS

Introduction   ix

Frequently Used Terms   xvii

CHAPTER 1   The Imaginary Husband   1

CHAPTER 2   Superman   11

CHAPTER 3   Jesus, My Boyfriend   23

CHAPTER 4   The Chads   35

CHAPTER 5   Anchor Men   45

CHAPTER 6   Peter Pans   61

CHAPTER 7   Mr. Maybe   71

CHAPTER 8   Jack Daniels   81

CHAPTER 9   The Critics   95

CHAPTER 10 Captain Vacationship   113

CHAPTER 11 Anchor Men Revisited   125

CHAPTER 12 The Doctor   137

CHAPTER 13 The Sages   149

CHAPTER 14 Dave the Watchmaker   163

CHAPTER 15 The Narrator   183

Acknowledgments   191

Notes   195

About the Author   206

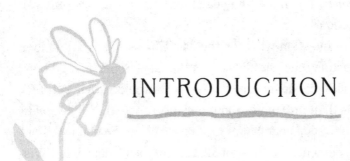

INTRODUCTION

The summer before I turned forty, I sat in the office of my somatic therapist, whom I'd been seeing for six months, and cried after purging details of my latest mistake, this time a one-night stand with a charming mustachioed boat captain in the Caribbean. Glenda, who I thought had surely tired of my tales, slowly looked up from her notes, held out her hands, and gently said, "Amanda, longing is your lover."

I sat still and silent, as one does when they've heard a hard truth that explains how they've navigated much of their life.

"You've been experiencing limerence," Glenda said.

Over twenty-five years, there must have been a hundred men—some encounters went no further than an exchange on an online dating app, some were exotic flings, some were ongoing "situationships" that burrowed deep into my heart for decades and strangled my ability to find real, committed love. Three I called my "Anchor Men"—not because they made me feel stable (quite the opposite) but because of how mired, or anchored, I felt in my own insecurities as a result of these back-to-back rejections.

Glenda was right. I was in love with longing, the anticipation of being desired, and the fear and grief of being rejected. My behavior seemed poetically described by the German word *Sehnsucht*, a combination of the words *das Sehnen*, meaning "the yearning," and *sucht*, meaning "an obsession or addiction."

I had begun to question whether the sacredness of sex I'd so long believed in was just as much an illusion as the false Supermen I'd been chasing—the narcissistic adventure runner who would rather run fifty miles in the woods than talk to me about our future together. The *almost* divorced man who would spend hours talking to me on the phone but put off meeting me in person. And most of all, the gorgeous, depressed Wisconsin farmer turned artist with whom I'd hook up with every couple years.

There were also nice guys, emotionally and physically available men who stood before me with their arms wide open, but I picked them apart like my grandma did a Thanksgiving turkey. I found flaws a metal detector couldn't find. I found the nice guys utterly boring, so I rejected them.

Psychologists call this mental state limerence, while the neuroscientists call it "person addiction." Taylor Swift sang about it in "Enchanted" and "Fortnight," and the troubadours of the Middle Ages chronicled limerence in their lyric poetry. Scarlett O'Hara was limerent for Ashley Wilkes in *Gone with the Wind*, and in *Love Actually*, Mark experiences limerence for Juliet, his best friend's wife. Limerence is ruminating (sometimes obsessively) about a romantic interest whom you've illogically placed on a pedestal (sans flaws)—someone who is just out of reach but for whom you have hope a relationship could develop.

In 1979, experimental psychologist Dorothy Tennov coined the term *limerence* in her book *Love and Limerence: The Experience of Being in Love*, which is based on a decade of research and several hundred case studies of romantic attachment.[1] Limerence produces the same euphoric feelings a person experiences in the first stages of love, so essentially it can happen to both people in an encounter. But the painful aspects of limerence may manifest as what's left over when those euphoric feelings linger for one person but not the other or as the secret longing for someone who may not even know you exist. Unlike erotomania, a cognitive state in which a person is delusional in thinking they are loved by and being pursued by the object of their love, those experiencing limerence feel deeply uncertain about whether the object of their desire will ever reciprocate their attention.

This longing for reciprocation is addictive and isolating at times. Someone experiencing limerence is constantly looking for signs of interest from the limerent object (LO) and deeply fears rejection. Any sign of interest feels euphoric, and any sign of rejection feels like grief. The limerent fantasy is usually not sexual in nature—it's more about a desire to be seen and cared for.[2] Limerence thrives when uncertainty mixes with a contest—can we win the LO's affection?—thus making hookup culture (a game based on status) the perfect fuel.

Some researchers, most notably Albert Wakin and Duyen Vo, argue limerence is a disorder ("an involuntary interpersonal state that involves intrusive, obsessive and compulsive thoughts, feelings, and behaviors"[3]) that belongs in the *Diagnostic and Statistical Manual of Mental Disorders* (*DSM*). Many see it as a result of having obsessive-compulsive disorder (OCD), attention deficit hyperactivity disorder (ADHD), and/or autism. When neuroscientist Dr. Tom Bellamy randomly surveyed more than fifteen hundred respondents, he found that more than 60 percent had experienced limerence.[4] Of those people, 50 percent said they'd had limerence so bad that it had disrupted their lives and caused borderline dysfunctional behavior. There was statistically no difference in occurrence between men and women.

As a late-in-life virgin, I had become paralyzed by an unsolvable equation: (How long to wait × How far to go) ÷ (How much love and commitment was enough). I worried my parameters around sex were keeping me from the relationship I was seeking.

Limerence, for me, was the perfect escape from real intimacy. However, it was disrupting my productivity at work, and it was also wasting my precious fertile time to have the child I deeply desired. It had damaged close friendships and blinded me to healthy relationships that were staring me in the face.

With most of my intense crushes, I found it therapeutic to write about them, almost as a way of documenting them to make the emotional energy and time invested count for something. I became obsessed with mentally completing experiences with men that had left me with scraps of an incomplete story. I could live for months, sometimes a year, on imagining the ending to these unresolved relationships. These men were my muses. They inspired research.

But there's no finish line for an endurance runner who keeps running herself in circles. And so I sought advice from a Japanese psychic, a consecrated virgin, a somatic therapist, a decision scientist, a rabbi and author on intimacy, and a former Chicago mobster turned addictions counselor. I spoke with psychologists studying limerence and attachment styles, neuroscientists studying romantic longing in the brain, and sociologists studying college hookup culture. I reached out to experts on grief, social psychologists who studied personality, and a renowned Buddhist mindfulness teacher. I interviewed men and women who found limerence had ruled their love life for decades. I read dozens of academic journal articles and interviewed some of the experts who had written them on my podcast, *The Longing Lab*. I pored over ten years' worth of emails from readers who recognized themselves in my essays on relationship struggles—women and men in the United States, Australia, India, Cameroon, Indonesia, France, England, Ireland, Hungary, and Brazil.

After a decade of research, I realized that a lot of the same cultural, psychological, and neurological factors that had encouraged my steadfast virginity were also influencing an ever-increasing number of other singles to get stuck in limerence—longing for the "fairy tale" relationship while chasing emotionally or physically unavailable individuals. I wanted that loving, committed relationship badly, but my ADHD brain was more attracted to the pattern of pursuing love with the goal of "winning" the unwinnable. It was safer than trying to receive love from someone who might reject me.

Longing for the ideal partner in the ideal location at the ideal time kept me distracted from my fear of making an imperfect decision—something I learned was an increasingly common fear in today's dating world, where dating apps and social media suggest perfect is possible if only you keep searching. Through research, I learned anticipation was my drug: It's not when we get what we want but when we anticipate it that the motivation molecule dopamine is released.

"Holding onto" my virginity had become a protective mechanism in a "sex positive" dating world that demands physical intimacy but admonishes emotional intimacy, where options seem plentiful but connections ambiguous. Like many of my Christian, Muslim, Sikh, and Jewish friends raised in faith-abiding households, I had to find a way in college to navigate a world where the "instructions" I was receiving were at odds with each other: how to be both "good" and "desired" and never settle for anything but the best. Limerence was a safe place to hide because it meant I could still fantasize about the men I was grinding with on the dance floor without actually crossing my boundaries.

Women growing up post–sexual revolution were raised to think we were free to chase our dreams—academic, athletic, professional, and even romantic. We were told we could have it all. There was even a name for us: the "alpha female." But when it came to dating, especially in a sea of non-committal men, this model often didn't work. Through limerent reverie, though, I could set a lofty goal of attaining idealized love. I could even imagine a successful outcome despite feeling left in limbo after an alcohol-fueled hookup—a casual sexual encounter (without intercourse, in my case).

I fell in love with strangers, men with whom I could never have full closure but could infinitely envision. And when my chase for an emotionally out-of-reach lover grew boring, I expanded my search to include Captain Vacationships—men who lived far away, often in exotic places. I chose dead-end paths with men who would quit me before I had the chance to quit them.

I have learned that part of healing is first observing our deep wounds. This requires self-compassion and recognizing the illusion of control. For so long, I tried to shame myself out of the perceived loss of a relationship. But, by practicing self-love, as both a feeling and a thinking skill, I could stop chasing love and learn to receive it from a man standing before me with his arms wide open.

Why This Book

If you find yourself collecting experiences with hot guys who leave you only breadcrumbs...

If you plan trips abroad in hopes of meeting your soulmate but ignore the nice guy next door ...

If you deeply fear settling for a partner who is less than perfect for you...

If you blow off friends or work to spend time immersed in your Netflix crush or book boyfriend...

If you have a mug that says "worthy of love" but don't believe it ...

If you've ever dog-eared copies of *Why Men Love Bitches* or clicked on the Facebook ad "How to Make Him Choose You" ...

If you've ever used ChatGPT to replace the human crush who is ghosting you ...

If you dissociate after using alcohol to numb yourself during intimacy...

If you're unhappily married and self-medicating with limerent fantasies of men online who praise you ...

If you find yourself attracting and then chasing after unavailable men because it's easier than risking accepting love from someone who might disappear...

I've written this book for you.

When Longing Becomes Your Lover is broken into three parts: (1) the seeds of limerence, (2) the mess of limerence, and (3) the emergence from limerence. Although I'm not a therapist or a scientist, I have experienced limerence for most of my life and spent years studying it as a journalist, linguist, and body worker. Woven into my personal journey throughout this book is academic research and my interviews with various experts. I also include my conversations with like-minded women and men who have faced roadblocks to emotional intimacy and who might have used abstinence to create a false sense of safety. *When Longing Becomes Your Lover* explains why we get stuck in patterns of longing, how it keeps us from getting into a healthy relationship, and what we can do to stop these patterns and set ourselves on a path that allows for more conscious decision-making.

In writing parts of this book over the past two decades, I wrote myself out of romantic longing and into the happy relationship I'd dreamed of for decades. This book is what I wish I had had to read as I was navigating the dating world and searching for a life partner. Whether you are single, married, or divorced, my hope is that *When Longing Becomes Your Lover* helps you better understand your patterns and provides ways you can improve your quest for love.

Some names, places, and physical characteristics have been changed to protect individuals' identities.

FREQUENTLY USED TERMS

Anchor Man: A past romantic flame who arrived in someone's life at a major transition time and whose rejection was emotionally crippling and, as a result, linked to self-defining memories

Glimmer: The specific characteristics (i.e., scents, physical traits, archetypes) of a limerent object that subconsciously spark limerence

Limerence: A state of mind in which one ruminates, sometimes obsessively, over a person of romantic interest in hopes of emotional reciprocation

Limerent: The person experiencing limerence

Limerent Object (LO): The individual who is often emotionally or physically unavailable that the limerent has placed on a pedestal

Limerent Supply: Anything that is fuel for limerence (memories, smells, social media, fantasy, photos, letters, etc.)

Love Bombing: A manipulative tactic, often used by narcissists, to lure or keep someone in a relationship through excessive flattery, passionate declarations of love, and/or over-the-top gifts

FREQUENTLY USED TERMS

Lover-Shadow: Originally coined by H.G. Wells, a vision of idealized love imagined as a child that shapes who we pursue and attach to later in life.

Purity Culture: A Christian movement in the nineties that encouraged young adults to remain sexually abstinent until marriage

Note: Some argue there are two types of limerence—romantic and non-romantic. My book focuses on the romantic kind.

CHAPTER 1

THE IMAGINARY HUSBAND

Everything that is real was imagined first.
—Margery Williams, *The Velveteen Rabbit*

While other five-year-olds were busy with imaginary friends, I had an imaginary husband named Dave the Watchmaker who went with me everywhere. I vividly recall my first wedding, where my mom played "The Bridal Chorus" on the organ as I walked down a makeshift aisle in our family living room carrying a giant plastic baby doll. Even when I was a child, there was something empowering about being able to make it all happen perfectly in my imagination. Dave the Watchmaker was reliable, a consistent plus-one for whatever events a five-year-old had to attend.

But why a watchmaker? Why not a fireman? Or a doctor? Or a chemist, like my dad? In one early episode of *Mister Rogers' Neighborhood* I'd watched as a four-year-old, a watchmaker took apart a watch to clean it. Perhaps this foreshadowed my attraction to men whose emotions seemed elusive—like they were a watch to take apart, examine, and fix. The clock tower was a central feature in the Land of Make Believe, and it would become one in my own life. Longing would become a misleading attempt at control, a crutch, when inevitably the clock kept ticking.

From a young age, before specifically romantic longing was even on my radar, I was a curious "longer"—someone who was always seeking something or somewhere outside myself to generate excitement, seeing connections where others saw none. But to an outsider looking at my childhood environment, my longing would have seemed odd. I had a good life. I grew up with supportive and loving parents, teachers, and friends in Fairfield, Ohio, a quiet suburb of Cincinnati. My parents were happily married high school sweethearts and professed to be each other's best friend. They modeled teamwork, forgiveness, and a growth mindset.

I was healthy. I had a room full of art supplies, Cabbage Patch Kids, Strawberry Shortcake figurines, and board games. We took trips to the zoo and amusement park. Whatever I showed interest in pursuing, my parents gave me the opportunity: ballet, swimming, acting, gardening, piano, writing, drawing, photography, and more.

As for many little girls, my father was my Prince Charming, a practical, selfless, and often emotionally reserved chemist dedicated first to his family and second to work. He was a calculated risk-taker and weary of bullshitters. As a first-grader, he'd left a note for Santa to officially sign on the dotted line to validate he was the one dropping off the presents. My aunt Marsha recalls my father the next day placing the paper in his safe, believing the signature might be worth something "when Santa was dead." He admittedly connected better with animals than with people. Hugs were few and far between, and when they happened, they were one-armed hugs. However, the tall dark brunet with big brown eyes showed his love through action: playing Wiffle ball in the backyard, helping me build elaborate forts, defrosting my car on winter mornings, and making sure I had the right vitamins.

He took me on practical father–daughter dates grounded in nature. We went driving and pulled off highways where the road drove through hills blown apart by dynamite and we scrambled up the sides in search of trilobite fossils and rocks that sparkled. We collected leaves at Harbin

Park and placed them on chromatography paper to let the sun bleach out the edges around them. We fished for bass and bluegill in the lakes of Ohio and Indiana. He took me for pony rides, and we refueled with donuts.

But despite knowing in my heart that my father deeply loved me, my head felt like I had to win his love and respect.

Maybe my restlessness was due to my Enneagram sign of 7 (known as "The Enthusiast") playing out at a young age—fearing boredom, chasing the next adventure, and pursuing new relationships—or maybe my astrological sign of Aquarius made me dream of fanciful ideas and places. Maybe it was just how my mind was naturally wired.

I wondered how much my seeking an extension of myself, my feeling of dislocation, stemmed from being separated from my mother as an infant for almost a month at birth. I'd almost lost my mother before I met her. Twenty minutes after the doctor pulled me out with forceps, my mother had a grand mal seizure that resulted from a blood vessel bursting in her brain. Ten minutes later, she had another.

"I don't know which hurt more: the labor pains or the pressure in my brain," my mom said.

"They kept you in the nursery for five days until they knew I would live," she told me when I was thirty-seven, describing the events following her cerebral hemorrhage. "Then your grandma Nancy took care of you for three weeks before I could leave the hospital. Grandma Velda was too traumatized by the situation to care for a newborn," my mom said, rolling her eyes. She'd always felt like her mom, Velda, was more of a needy burden than a help. Grandma Nancy, like her son (my father), was adept at suppressing her feelings and needs to deal with the task at hand.

"The nurse told Dad she'd seen mothers go home without their babies, but in thirty years of work, you were the first baby to go home without its mother," my mother said. It would be three weeks before my mother could return home to me and six weeks before she felt like mothering. I can't imagine how hard this must have been for her, a natural caretaker. I've known her to find homes for stray dogs, offer extended shelter and care to her medically compromised students, and become the legal guardian of an elderly woman with no family.

My mother's retelling of our birth story is a legend in which she plays both victim and martyr. For twenty days (five of which she couldn't hold me), she had to lie flat on her back drugged with morphine. Then she was sent home to tend to her firstborn during an ice storm that actually cut the electricity for three days.

When my mother would tell me the story, often my father would sigh and leave the room. He clearly did not want to relive the events of her aneurysm and her seemingly miraculous recovery—the only reason, he says, he believes in God to this day.

When I asked my mother why—why a blood vessel burst in her brain—she laughed. "You kept going in and out and in and out of the birth canal—couldn't make up your mind then, can't make it up now." The truth I'd learn as an adult was that my mother was pushing while holding her breath, but this tale of my own poor decision-making was the story I was repeatedly told as I was growing up.

It was my fault, I concluded.

Although we don't consciously remember these traumas at birth, I always wondered how much time an infant spent separated from their birth mother was too much time. Was my grandma Nancy's attention enough? Psychology research shows an infant's separation from its mother for as short as one week causes "neurobiological vulnerability" like the insecure/disorganized attachment style I exhibited later in life.[1]

When experimental social psychologist Dorothy Tennov began her research in the seventies on what she'd call "limerence," she was laying the groundwork for attachment theory. Over the next couple decades, attachment theory research took off and limerence got left in the dust. However, recent researchers of limerence note how childhood post-traumatic stress disorder (CPTSD) or microtraumas (small, repeated acts that accumulate over time to create long-lasting emotional wounds) plant the seeds for limerence later in life. These inner childhood wounds come in the form of abandonment, questioned worth, rejection, and neglect. For some limerents I spoke with, their limerence resulted from growing up with a parent with alcoholism, narcissism, and/or depression. Others described traumas related to sexual abuse, parental divorce, adoption, or frequent moving from one town to another. Many can't pinpoint any one trauma.

Recent research notes how having ADHD and/or autism can make one more likely to develop limerent tendencies (and be more sensitive to rejection).[2] In his book *Scattered Minds*, renowned addiction expert Dr. Gabor Maté attributes ADHD to childhood trauma, including separation at birth.[3] It's easy to connect the dots. If trauma at birth can lead to developing ADHD and ADHD makes one more likely to experience limerence, then it makes sense that, as early as third grade, I would be hyperfocused on romantic interests that felt familiar and similar to that out-of-reach maternal love I'd longed for as an infant. In her book *Mother Hunger*, therapist Kelly McDaniel describes this "invisible heartache."[4]

Freudian psychoanalytic theory suggests that our first longing is for our mother in her absence. Analysts believe that as young children we develop a "Lover-Shadow" that shapes who we pursue or form attachments with in our future as an adult. "One might say that the wishful fantasy of a loving figure may be all the stronger for having had to be imagined," writes renowned psychoanalyst Ethel Person in her 1988 book *Dreams of Love and Fateful Encounters*.[5]

I wondered if my imaginary husband Dave the Watchmaker resembled my Lover-Shadow?

Emotional Dysregulation: You're Too Much

My mother was determined to raise me with more affection and concern than she'd experienced as an often lonely only child. But when I was three, I began having episodes of strange behavior—or "fits," as my mother refers to them—that concerned my parents. My mother was a double major in speech pathology and early childhood education, but I presented a case she hadn't studied. Confused and exasperated, she described my behavior to the pediatrician as irrational and stubbornly defiant. Applying a diagnosis that the medical community no longer uses, the pediatrician suggested my parents put me on medication to treat "psychomotor seizures." The name the pediatrician used for my "seizures" (with no apparent convulsions) described a temporary impairment of consciousness characterized by psychic symptoms (visual and auditory hallucinations and déjà vu), loss of judgment, and abnormal acts.

Thankfully, my parents opted to take me to a neurologist instead of accepting the drugs. After examining me and reading my mom's journal tracking my behavior, the neurologist stated I was the "brightest and most strong-willed preschooler" she'd ever encountered. She laughed and wished them luck. Nonmedical diagnosis: I was an independent little girl with a vivid imagination. In my mind, if I could dream it, I could will it to come true. A doctor today might look at me as a preschooler with "exaggerated" emotional responses, distractibility, anxiety, a tendency to daydream and be self-critical and suggest I had ADHD (a diagnosis I wouldn't receive until I was thirty-six years old).

Longing + Imagination = Escape

I was obsessed with Dorothy Gale—America's heartland princess who believed in traveling "Over the Rainbow" in search of fulfilling her heart's desire. The song—what I'd later learn was called the "I Want" song in musicals and Disney movies—became my personal anthem.

Every February, right around my birthday, I became Dorothy Gale. I sat with my stuffed Toto dog and picnic basket watching the annual telecast of *The Wizard of Oz*. I identified with Dorothy and dreamed of "somewhere" over the rainbow—somewhere better, if not magical. Somewhere in Technicolor. Somewhere, perhaps the source of the divine.

When I was five, I began threatening to run away from home. Only once did I make it past the front porch. But, after multiple threats, my father, tired of my games, actually began offering to help me pack my bag.

What I wanted (but didn't realize then) was to be found.

I learned to channel my defiant energy into creating adventures where there was none to be had. I did the "Over the Rainbow" kind of dreaming with a little belief in magic (something Grandma Velda thought sinful).

I determined the forest behind my house (home to a 150-year-old unkempt graveyard) was magical. I hiked friends back to the "Cavern of Wilderness" for pretend séances. We'd dare each other to stand on top of moss-covered graves hidden under a canopy of overgrown vines and make wishes.

As young as nine, I connected romance with the exotic, somewhere far away where magic seemed to have a better chance. Young enough to still sit on Santa's lap, but old enough to know the myth of Santa, I asked Santa for a boyfriend from Florida—the home of Disney, where I'd *heard* dreams came true. I'd grown up on Disney's most limerent fantasy: the Little Mermaid—a girl who gives up her voice for the chance to meet the guy she fell in love with at first sight. Santa responded, "I'll see what I can do."

In sixth grade, when friends began coupling up at our first middle school dances and my friend Lynn and I were already bemoaning singlehood, we developed another world called "No-Man-Land." Our slam book stories referenced the "Seas of Singlehood," "Rivers of Retreat," and "Islands of Isolation" found on the map we'd spent days drawing. It was our own paracosm, a community with its own distinctive geography and history.

Forget the ancient divination tool of plucking daisy petals. On sleepovers, we'd pull out the Ouija board and try to conjure up answers to our deepest questions. "Will Josh ask me to sit with him on the bus?" We dreamed about our future playing the fortune-telling game MASH on paper, where we'd make our list of five in each category (men, job, car, number of children, place of residence, etc.) and then cross them off one by one according to our chosen number until our fate was decided.

In seventh grade, I devoured my first romance novel, which I'd picked up in the used books section of the town library. *Albuquerque*, by Sara Orwig, was a love affair between Noah McCloud, a long, dark-haired Confederate soldier, and bodice-bound April Danby. Historical western romance novels became my limerence porn, and their steamy passages were the first thing to physically arouse me as I read them curled up in my bedroom corner with the door closed. The passion and perfection in those love stories scratched the itch in the part of me that was intense and idealistic. I even began writing my own romance titled "Forget Me Not."

Back then, *BORE* was the worst possible four-letter word. My mom would say, "Every day has to be a circus for you, doesn't it?!" when I'd complain of being miserably bored (another ADHD trait). I had some unsatisfied yearning for being somewhere bigger and better than where I was. At a young age, I was pursuing the pleasure felt in anticipation.

Longing for "Home"

One popular thread on Reddit describes limerence as "being homesick for a place that only exists in your mind."[6] *Home* is a place or a time or a person where or when or with whom we can be ourselves and still feel unconditionally loved. *Heaven*, *home*, and *love* all become synonymous.

As soon as I was old enough to read, I sang, "Be Thou my Dignity, Thou my Delight; Thou my soul's Shelter, Thou my high Tower," from hymnal books while standing in a pew with peers and family. I believed in my heart "'Tis grace hath brought me safe thus far, And grace will lead me home." These were songs and expressions I sang and whose words I knew by heart. The Christian messages I grew up on in Sunday school and vacation Bible school encouraged me to long for my heavenly home and that promised partner. I was told God had a plan, and I believed it. I was eleven when Madonna released her hit single "Like a Prayer" in which she sings about someone calling her name and how that feels like home. Who is calling her? A lover? A place? God?

The English word *longing* just doesn't capture the intense highs and lows I felt in my youth for people, places, and time. The Portuguese word *saudade* comes close: a melancholic or profoundly nostalgic longing for someone or something that is long gone or that may have never existed. And the Russian word *toska* comes closer. Vladimir Nabokov described it as "a sensation of great spiritual anguish, often without any specific cause. At less morbid levels it is a dull ache of the soul, a longing with nothing to long for, a sick pining, a vague restlessness, mental throes, yearning. In particular cases it may be the desire for somebody or some-thing specific, nostalgia, lovesickness."[7]

Was I born with some knowing of the past for which I yearned?[8] A past life? The researchers Lynn Willmott and Evie Bentley link limerence with "an inclination to reintegrate unresolved past life(s) experiences and to progress to a state of greater authenticity (i.e., being truer to one's inner self)."[9] There's something about longing that satisfies a desire to connect with a different time—any time but the ennui of the present.

Passionate Children

The year I was born (1978), psychologist Elaine Hatfield would define passionate love as "a state of intense longing for a union with another."[10] In the mid-eighties, Hatfield developed the Juvenile Love Scale, based on her team's Passionate Love Scale, as a way to examine the emotional, behavioral, and cognitive indicators suggesting a "longing for love" in children and young adolescents (ages 3 to 18).[11]

The assessment asks children to imagine a person who gets them very excited who meets the characteristics of a "crush." Then the children rate their answers to fifteen questions on a nine-point scale, from *agree very little* (1) to *agree very much* (9). The questions are like these: "Did you ever keep thinking about _____ when you wanted to stop and couldn't?" and "I want to know all I can about _____." And "If I could, when I grow up, I'd like to marry/live with _____."

Individual scores are summed and interpreted as:

106–135 points = Wildly, recklessly in love

86–105 points = Passionate but less intense

66–85 points = Occasional bursts of passion

45–65 points = Tepid, infrequent passion

15–44 points = The thrill is gone

I'm sure I would've scored "wildly" high on Hatfield's scale. Though Dave the Watchmaker faded away before I entered elementary school, the groundwork was laid for romantic longing for seemingly out-of-reach crushes, albeit visible ones.

As early as third grade, I was practicing "light" limerence. Friends just called me a hopeless romantic. Like many preteens, I had celebrity crushes and wrote hopeful letters to the eighties TV star Kirk Cameron. I was the awkward, nerdy girl crushing on Josh, the most popular boy in our third-grade class, and envisioning the moment when he would come to his senses and fall in love with me. I got a thrill out of riding my bike past his house in hopes and fear he might see me. The tension was exhilarating—and sometimes debilitating.

In further research, Elaine Hatfield and her colleagues found in adolescents a significant correlation between experiencing anxiety and experiencing passionate love.[12]

One afternoon in fifth grade, I lay on the couch sobbing after hearing that my new crush named Bryan liked my friend. My chest was tight, and I felt like I was breathing through a straw. "Hun, don't cry," my grandma Velda called from the kitchen as she cut handmade noodles for dinner. She was an Illinois-raised farm girl born during the 1918 Spanish flu pandemic and raised in the Depression. She clipped coupons and used straws because she didn't trust the cleanliness of restaurant glasses. She moved in with us when I was eight and often helped with cooking, cleaning, and watching over my brother and me while my parents were at work. Despite my young age, we confided in each other things we didn't tell my mother (like the time the chiropractor kissed Grandma).

"There will be plenty more," she said about Bryan, trying to reassure me.

Much to her dismay, there would be way more than she'd prayed for me to ever have.

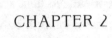

CHAPTER 2

SUPERMAN

Flying is the biological taboo of our species. Humans are land creatures who can walk, run, swim, but cannot fly. Except in our dreams, we are forbidden from entering that Eden. So it's small wonder that we long for the forbidden gift, that we crave flight, and imagine our gods waltzing across the sky.

—Diane Ackerman, *A Natural History of Love*

Freudian psychoanalysts believe we spend decades searching for the idealized composite of a lover we imagined as children. This sought-after Lover-Shadow has what psychologists call a unique "glimmer" (the distinct personal qualities we've prioritized) that hooks us. In our imaginations, we transform our love interests, namely by overlooking their flaws, so that they embody the Lover-Shadow that lives in our psyche.

Writers—with no psychology training—described this phenomenon centuries ago. In his book *On Love*, nineteenth-century French writer Stendhal (Marie-Henri Beyle) wrote, "You have conceived an ideal without knowing it. . . . One day you come across someone not unlike this idea;

11

crystallization . . . consecrates forever to the master of your destiny what you have dreamt of for so long." Here Stendhal describes the moment of crystallization in limerence, the moment when the limerent object is idealized, a century before Dorothy Tennov even coined the term *limerence*. Like a bare rock bedazzled with gems, the ordinary guy (in my case) became extraordinary after crystallization.[1]

Perhaps the seed for the idealized hero was planted on nights when I was five and got to stay up late enough to watch *The Greatest American Hero*. Or perhaps it was when I binge-watched *The Boy Who Could Fly* on the VHS tape my church friend Bella gifted me for my eleventh birthday. I was enamored with the tale of a high school girl who reaches and seemingly rescues the autistic boy next door, who in turn takes her flying. They fall in love, but the essential piece of the story is: He then disappears. It set the stage for my soon-to-blossom obsession with unattainable relationships with men who themselves needed rescuing.

In my early junior high years, I developed faith in a culturally contrived vision of Superman: the mysterious hero, the wait, the rescue, and the surrender. Christopher Reeve's *Superman* movie, arguably the most popular of the Superman series, was released the year I was born. Although I wouldn't see the film until junior high, it shaped me. The features of Reeve's face were burned into my memory as a model of perfection. In high school, I binge-watched *Somewhere in Time* in which Reeve's character, playwright Richard Collier, uses self-hypnosis to travel seventy years back in time to visit an actress whose photo he's fallen madly in love with. Like most serial limerents, I would become very good at mental time travel in the form of replaying conversations or moments of eye contact with my LOs.

Songs that idolized the concept of a Superman figure, someone who would rescue me from my boring but safe trajectory, fed my obsession: Pat Benatar's "I Need a Hero!" Mariah Carey's "Hero," and Crash Test Dummies' "Superman." I was only eight years old when I heard Peter Cetera sing, "I'll be the hero you're dreaming of." During fourth-grade indoor recess, we listened over and over to Belinda Carlisle's hit single "Heaven Is a Place on Earth" on my best friend Mallory's ghetto blaster. During church services, I sang, "I am weak, you are strong" and "Jesus rescues me." On bus trips to the local amusement park, our driver would blast megachurch Hillsong's "Jesus Is My Superhero."

Perfectionism

The process of imagining my LOs into the ideal hero was cerebrally appealing to me. As the oldest grandchild and the older sibling to a brother who struggled, I felt I had to strive for perfection. My maternal line was full of world-champion perfectionists.

Psychologist and author of *Loving Bravely* and *Love Every Day*, Dr. Alexandra Solomon, explained it to me this way: "Often the oldest daughter develops perfectionism because there's this expectation of her to be the good girl—to be successful. And there's a way that achievement and goodness serve a function for the family." Solomon, who draws from family systems theory for her research, admits she filled the perfectionist role in her family.

"If we feel that we're expected to excel and we're female, then I think that pulls towards romantic stories, you know, idealized love. Straight A's are one way of tapping into that achievement, but this draw towards perfect love makes sense too," Solomon explained.[2]

Goals

There's a reason my friends called me "Flavor of the Month" by the time I got to high school—I'd had back-to-back crushes with scant relationships between. A new crush meant a new rush. In sixth grade, I was laser-focused on the blond-haired, blue-eyed neighborhood hottie two years older than me who cut our lawn and delivered newspapers. I fantasized about him casting me a flirty wink even though he had no clue I watched him as he mowed the backyard. In eighth grade, it was the big-eyed kid on the swim team who went to the private Catholic school in town. Occasionally, he'd flirt with me, tugging at my feet when he'd swim by. But then he'd ignore me at the pool wall. He was the first guy whose mixed messages had me on the hook. And, ultimately, he'd be my first date—a Sunday night out with his Catholic youth group.

As an athlete who filled her calendar with competitions, I sought out goals to achieve. In a like manner, I couldn't stop liking one boy until I had another crush lined up; otherwise, my ADHD brain would feel itchy. It needed a limerent object on which to hyperfocus to generate that dopamine my brain was lacking.[3] This pattern was an energetic organizing force for me. I was becoming what psychologists call "serially limerent," with a few long-lasting limerent crushes thrown in for "sustainability," I suppose. My life's timeline was delineated by crushes.

The average onset of the first limerent episode among those who go on to be serially limerent is fifteen years old.[4] Although some, like clinical social worker Brandy Wyant, have documented episodes of limerence occurring as early as childhood. In her published clinical self-study, Wyant reported a history of limerent episodes starting as early as four years of age. For her, they were platonic longings for another female she idolized.[5] My LOs were always romantic interests in males who became elusive goals to pursue.

As for many limerents, my intense crushes lasted only about a year, maybe two. But the first long-lasting LO would creep into my dreams and stay there for almost two decades. I met Sam in church youth group the summer before my freshman year in high school. The blond-haired, blue-eyed six-foot-two pillar was already entering his sophomore year, so as an older man and one my grandma praised, he felt like a formidable challenge for me.

That year at school, with a little encouragement from my mom, I asked him to Homecoming, and, to my bewilderment, he agreed. The night of the dance, I shook with so much anxiety I rarely took off the little red bolero my grandma had sewn for me. I would berate myself for years to come for allowing my anxiety to turn me stiff as a board that night.

Junior year in high school, I went on a "mission" trip with five guys (including Sam) and our youth group leader to Illinois to help residents clean up after a flood. My only "mission" was getting Sam to fall in love with me.

"You haven't seen anything until you've seen Sam with his shirt off," I'd told Grandma Velda one Sunday after admiring his perfect pecs at a youth group pool party. The following Sunday in the church sanctuary as I stood next to Sam, she approached us with a wide grin. I shot her a "don't you dare" look, already mortified of what I saw coming. She asked Sam to take his shirt off, and then she proceeded to tell him what I'd said. He nervously chuckled, but his shirt remained firmly gripping his pecs.

For four years, I went to church to see him. I dressed for church to see him. I went to church youth group events to see him. I managed to sit through boring sermons by staring at Sam, envisioning him kissing me. I silently schemed ways I might get to spend time with him after church. I'd position myself during prayer in hopes we might all be asked to bow our heads and hold hands; I'd hope he'd take his shirt off during volleyball matches in our youth leader's backyard; I'd sit near him on bus rides to events and listen to him share racy stories from church camp. Any smirk or glance from him I took as a glimmer of hope for our future together.

For his graduation, I made an arrangement with the teacher in charge of line leaders so that I could lead his row during the ceremony. And when he was deployed overseas in the military, I sent him letters and care packages. The few times he wrote back or the one time he called on Christmas Eve, my heart leapt. The theme song for my crush on Sam was Linda Ronstadt's "Long, Long Time" and I listened to it on repeat. It felt good to ache for someone.

Impossible Relationships

I binge-watched *Pretty Woman*'s Vivian Ward (Julia Roberts) wrestle with her childhood fantasy. Vivian, a prostitute, declares she wants the fairy tale when her love interest millionaire Edward Lewis (Richard Gere) asks her how much more she wants. Later in the film, Edward declares that his "special gift is impossible relationships." Like Edward and Vivian, my gift was imagining I could make the impossible come true. It would take me years to realize that any idealized relationship is an impossible relationship.

As a sophomore, I became obsessed with a senior, No. 32 on the basketball team. This dark-haired, blue-eyed star jock was almost as out of reach as Superman, but I knew where he parked his car and where he'd be after third period. I'd walk past his locker as he flirted with a pretty blonde from the soccer team and get the weak-knees high that would send me back again the next day. Even the slightest brush up against him and whiff of his deodorant in our sardine-packed hallways renewed my hope, as if through osmosis I had been transferred his affection. Mallory's sister's boyfriend played basketball with No. 32 and clued us in on where he lived, so Mallory and I would occasionally drive by his house hoping he might be outside shooting hoops.

For my sixteenth birthday, a church friend arranged for No. 32 to deliver a red rose to me outside the cafeteria (out of sight from anyone—I presumed were his conditions). He was kind, maybe even a bit embarrassed himself, and wished me a happy birthday. I acted like one of those Beatlemania girls from the black-and-white films—but I didn't scream. After No. 32 walked away, I crumbled to the floor outside the doors of the cafeteria alone and sobbed—the kind of sobbing one does when deeply grieving the loss of someone dear to them. I was playing a game I could neither win nor lose. As Simone de Beauvoir says in her book *The Second Sex* in the chapter "The Woman in Love": "If she wins the game, she destroys her idol; if she loses it, she loses herself. There is no salvation."[6]

I felt heartbroken over a love story that existed only in my head.

In limerence, along with the high of imagining our crush interested in us comes a deep fear of rejection. To disclose your obsession to your crush could potentially destroy any hope. After all, limerence thrives on uncertainty. That is what that red rose scene entailed—the bubble burst. No. 32 knew. I replayed that scene over and over, searching for any sign that this mighty crush might just think I was worthy of his attention. Did our eyes lock like I thought they had? Did we brush hands? Did he stay longer than he had to?

Musical Direction

Living in limerence means you're on a treasure hunt every day looking for clues below a murky surface and connecting them to create meaning where it may not exist. My brain was super associative, so this process came naturally.

As a perfectionist who put a great burden on myself to make everything work on my own, I found great relief in following clues that someone (God or the universe) provided. One major clue I relied on for inspiration and direction on my treasure hunts was music. If I heard Led Zepplin's "Stairway to Heaven" or Van Halen's "Dreams," I immediately fell into reverie about Sam, as those were some of the songs he played in his car when he'd drive me to our youth group leader's house. Time after time, I made decisions based on what music happened to come on the radio.

What I didn't know then was how much the music was neurolinguistically shaping me. In one University of Toronto study, psychologists coded over eight hundred *Billboard* number one hits for their attachment themes. For songs from 1946 to 2015, they found that lyrics have become more avoidant and less secure over time.[7] This reflects social disconnection, which is a catalyst for longing. The more we listen to songs with distrusting lyrics, the more we distrust others. And the more I listened to lyrics expressing uncertainty and attachment anxiety, the more I felt unworthy of the hero I sought. Was I drawn to certain music because of my anxious avoidant attachment style or was the music shaping my attachment style? I don't know, but I do believe this increase in insecure lyrics sparked limerence in my generation and the ones to follow.

But it wasn't just my own generation's music I adored. I relished the Gershwin and Big Band tunes that romanticized anticipation, too.

Gramps played these songs, like "Someone to Watch over Me," on cassette tapes in his car. I believed I was not alone on my mission—someone out there wanted to be my hero, and he was meant to be.

Soulmates

It was my insightful Japanese high school exchange student friend and teammate Yumi who introduced me to the "Three Supermen" concept she grew up believing in Japan. During one training run, she told me that there are three possible soulmates out there for each person. You may never meet all three. You may meet the other two after you've married the first. Timing, timing, timing.

In his 2005 short story "The Kidney-Shaped Stone That Moves Every Day," Haruki Murakami illustrates this theory through the sixteen-year-old character Junpei and his father. "Among the women a man meets in his life, there are only three who have real meaning for him. No more, no less," his father said—or, rather, declared. "You will probably become involved with many women in the future," his father continued, "but you will be wasting your time if a woman is the wrong one for you."[8] My goodness, the pressure!

Then there was also the Japanese legend of destined love that claims we are all born with a red string of fate (known as Akai Ito) tied to our finger, and somewhere out there our string is connected to our soulmate's finger. My cynical side wondered how many soulmates had lost a finger by unknowingly straying too far from their destined love.

In the foundational work of Jewish mystical literature, Zohar, "twin souls are predestined before birth to reunite in matrimony."[9] God rejoins the souls, one male and one female. This matching, however, requires virtuous deeds to be committed by those reunited. In both Jewish and Christian texts, God, or Yahweh, is the Israelites' soulmate. The Yiddish word for destined partner is *bashert*.

As described in Plato's *Symposium*, Greek playwright Aristophanes tells a tale how once upon a time we were two souls connected in one body, so powerful in our oneness that Zeus broke us apart. Now we devote our lives to longing for and searching for our missing half—our twin flame.

Of the nearly fifteen thousand US adults interviewed in a 2021 YouGov poll, 60 percent of respondents said they believe in the idea of soulmates.[10] In a 2025 study, funded by Match.com and conducted in association with the Kinsey Institute, 69 percent of the five thousand US singles (ages 18–98) surveyed said they believe in destiny.[11] Those numbers surpass the percentage of Americans who believe in a biblical God (56 percent).[12]

In a recent BBC interview, Skidmore associate professor of religion Bradley Onishi discussed the innate nature of longing for a soulmate. "The soulmate myth promises fulfilment. It says that the isolation and loneliness that are so often part of the human experience are only temporary—that someday there will be a happily ever after in which we are united with The One who understands us at every level, protects us from harm and gives our life overwhelming significance," he told the BBC.[13] In other words, today's unpredictable dating culture is a catalyst for believing in a soulmate. It allows an individual to create a hopeful narrative in the midst of uncertainty and disappointment.

University of Houston professor of psychology Raymond Knee and colleagues say that our mental models of what makes a good or bad relationship shape how we approach dating and how we respond to challenges within relationships. People with what's called "destiny beliefs" are constantly evaluating their partner or potential partner to see if they measure up to the vision of their perfect match. Experts say this "alternative-seeking" behavior makes relationships fragile and sometimes even difficult to initiate.[14]

Others have "growth beliefs," which are built on the idea that great relationships develop over time and take two people working together to overcome problems. While those with high destiny beliefs ask, "Is this partner making me happy?" those with high growth beliefs ask, "What can we do together to strengthen our relationship?" In Knee's study, people with high growth beliefs were more likely to date someone for a long period of time, whereas those with high destiny beliefs were more likely to have one-night stands.

For most of high school, I was the destiny belief girl whose one-night stands existed only in her head, unless you consider my bouncing from crush to crush as one-night stands. By my senior year, I embodied the role of Lois in my Superman narrative. I can now see how I'd developed a borderline parasocial relationship with the movie. I started giving the name "Lane" to the hostesses who put me on waiting lists. I named my '87 Chevrolet Nova "Lois." I had a Superman keychain, bedroom poster, stickers, pens, stationery, watch, earrings, boxers, underwear, Christmas ornament, bumper sticker, and mug (to name a few). I had Lois Lane glasses. I dreamed of being a journalist.

Sure, everyone has their celebrity crushes and childhood idols. However, the extent to which I fantasized about a perfect hero distanced me in a way that made me highly critical of the nice guys who were interested in me.

After months of Mallory and I practicing kissing on our hands, I got my first kiss the week of my sixteenth birthday. Mark was not much over five foot five and had a soft, boyish body and matching immature humor. Upon dropping me off at home, Mark made his move (all while, unbeknownst to me, a handheld tape recorder in the glove box recorded his words). Celine Dion sang "The Power of Love" on the cassette player as he pulled into my driveway. My hand clenched the door handle as he professed his love. He leaned over and pressed his damp, slightly open mouth and then tongue to my tightly closed lips. I let it last a few seconds and then darted out the door with a quick, "Thanks!" When I slammed the front door and uttered a sound of disgust, my father yelled from the family room where he sat with my mom, "Scope is upstairs!"

The next morning at church, I learned that Mark had met with Sam after our date to play the recording of his declaration, what little there was. I felt like a pawn in their game. This first kiss, something I had dreamed being ecstasy at its best (and at the very least, deeply connecting), felt wasted on someone I found mediocre. I wouldn't make the mistake of settling again.

On Sunday nights of my senior year, you'd find me glued to the television series *Lois & Clark: The New Adventures of Superman*. "He's out there!" my grandma would assure me. Two weeks after they married, my grandmother waited for twenty-two months for her husband to return from World War II. To me, she defined a waiting to be revered, a steadfast faith.

CHAPTER 3

JESUS, MY BOYFRIEND

You will seek me and find me when you seek me with
all your heart.

—Jeremiah 29:13 (NIV)

My purity ring, not real gold, is now slightly bent. Fake diamonds outline an infinity symbol. It's housed in a small wooden jewelry box where I keep jewelry I'd want saved from a fire: my grandma Velda's pinkie ring, the Claddagh friendship ring from Yumi, my grandma Nancy's ruby-studded ring. In my thirties, my parents admitted they figured I would lose the purity ring, so they didn't invest much.

They'd always been open with me about sex. When I was in sixth grade, my mother gave me Peter Mayle's book about puberty titled *What's Happening to Me?* It was only then that I learned that I had a third hole down there. When I asked if the male sperm reached the vagina through a tube connecting the man and the woman, she explained how the anatomy actually functioned. "You do that with Dad?!" I asked, half disgusted and half in disbelief. "Yes, at least once a week," she responded confidently. For at least a week, I couldn't make eye contact with my father.

When I was about sixteen, I stood up in front of my church with other youth group friends pledging a vow of celibacy until we each were married. We sang Bryan Duncan's "Love Takes Time" and signed a pledge card I later stashed somewhere in my scrapbook. It said, "Believing that True Love Waits, I make a commitment to God, myself, my family, my friends, my future mate, and my future children to be sexually abstinent from this day until the day I enter a Biblical marriage relationship."[1]

Standing beside me was Bella, who (unbeknownst to me) had already lost her virginity as a freshman. She'd put herself on such a short leash after high school that she didn't even kiss the guy she married until her wedding day. On the other side stood Mark and Sam, snickering. In front of me stood Erica. She'd already had sex with her high school boyfriend, which our youth leader made her confess to her parents. She was also hiding the fact she'd been sexually abused in elementary school, but she hid that secret from her family until she was in her twenties. Years later, she'd tell me how she felt an indescribable longing she subconsciously suppressed through two ring ceremonies and marrying a man. When Erica was in her late twenties, she understood this longing was to be with another woman. The suppressed longing physically manifested in her body as "can't ride in the car" IBS and incredible weight gain. Hearing all this twenty years later on the phone with her made me sick to my stomach.

In the audience sat my parents, my brother, and my very proud grandma Velda. Her letters to me, addressed to her "precious Amanda" throughout my teens and twenties, were peppered with "Be a good girl" and "God has been good to you, but he may stop."

The scripture Grandma Velda wrote on index cards and I posted on my bulletin board assured me that, if I waited long enough and trusted him (not necessarily my gut), God's divine plan would unfold. Jeremiah 29:11 encouraged me: "For I know the plans I have for you," declares the Lord, "plans to prosper you and not to harm you, plans to give you hope and a future" (NIV). And Proverbs 3:5–6 reminded me: "Trust in the Lord with all your heart, and do not lean on your own understanding" (ESV). And then there was the promise from Psalm 37:4: "Delight yourself in the Lord and He will give you the desires of your heart" (ESV). The verses reinforced longing for a divinely appointed soulmate and eroticized waiting.

At the purity pledge ceremony, my father didn't creepily walk me down the aisle as I've heard happens in other churches. In fact, my parents didn't pressure me to pledge. Of course, not doing it would've made me an outcast among my peers, but it was also something I felt empowered to do. At the time, I believed in my mind, not yet in my gut, that sex was spiritually sacred, something to long for. I believed there was a calling, an ideal to quest for and then surrender to. I didn't realize it at the time, but this ceremony was fertilizer for my already seeded limerence. It would take two decades after I signed that pledge before science would prove what I felt to be true: Through orgasmic meditation studies, Dr. Andrew Newberg and colleagues would find that MRI brain scans depict an overlap in the brain between sexual ecstasy and spiritual ecstasy.[2]

And it wouldn't be until college that I'd witness in person the grandeur that is Gian Lorenzo Bernini's erotic sculpture *Ecstasy of Saint Teresa* in the Cornaro Chapel in Rome. The sixteenth-century nun reported in her autobiography, *The Life of Teresa of Jesus*, that an angel on fire visited her in her sleep at the age of forty-five and struck her heart with his golden spear. God, I yearned for that mystical, orgasmic, borderline tragic experience, but I didn't want to wait till I was forty-five!

Just before the ceremony, the boys and girls were split into groups to discuss the sanctity of sex and all the scary stuff—pregnancy, sexually transmitted infections, and, the worst, heartache. A female nurse in the congregation spoke to our group. I don't remember anything she said except her suggesting that, if we felt aroused, to masturbate with a zucchini or a carrot.

The church leaders, our youth minister, and our youth group leaders presented us with an exoskeleton of sexual ethics—hard and rigid. Truth with a capital T. This contrasted greatly with the endoskeleton of sexual ethics I'd later learn, a spine of values that changed depending on the scenario.

In Sunday school, sex was defined as penile penetration of a vagina. There were no variations of what "counted" and what didn't. As I gathered experiences and years, I had questions for those church leaders I wouldn't have dared ask even if I'd thought of them as a teen. Did failing the pledge mean never finding a future mate? Never having children (or more than one)? What about having oral sex? What about fingers? Masturbation? And did this contract have to remain in effect well into my thirties after most of my peers had already coupled up and the only singles left were used to having sex within the first five dates? Could you regrow your virginity, and if so, how long would it take? What was a "biblical marriage" anyways? What if I married someone of a different religion who still believed in God? Did engagement count? What if you were raped? And what if you never gave consent but felt saying no would ruin your chances of getting into a relationship with a man you were fixated on?

"Jesus Is My Boyfriend" Music

The worship music at church and on Christian radio echoed in words what Disney had provided in visuals: faith, longing, love, surrender, rescue, and happily ever after. I can still hear my grandma singing, "I come," as she gazed at the cross above the baptismal font. All the while, I quietly tripped over the lyrics and mentally undressed Sam of the perfectly formed pecs who stood three pews ahead of me.

The pop Christian artists of the nineties and early aughts wrote lyrics that blurred the lines between romantic love and Godly love. Songs like "I Could Sing of Your Love Forever," by Hillsong, is borderline limerent, and Amy Grant's "I Will Remember" romanticizes nostalgia and grief.

In Life House's hit single "Hanging by a Moment," they profess to be chasing and falling in love with "you." Jesus or someone else? Phil Wickham even titled a song "Divine Romance." In "How He Loves," the David Crowder Band speaks of heaven (Jesus?) meeting Earth like a "sloppy wet kiss." Kari Jobe's "The More I Seek You" describes a physically intimate relationship with Jesus, including drinking from his hands and feeling his heart beat. It's so overwhelming she wants to melt in his presence. Sounds like the kind of romance I was seeking.

But the "Jesus is my boyfriend" language was downright confusing.

Dr. Shannan Baker at Dunn Center for Christian Music Studies at Baylor University studies the connection between contemporary worship music and the practice of the church. "From what I've seen, I think the problem is when you start to hope that what you're singing to Jesus or asking from God can be fulfilled by anyone. When you start to look for perfect love, outside of the one who is perfect love, you're not gonna find it," she told me.[3]

This music was a limerent perfectionist high achiever's anthem. Set forth a noble challenge, and I would doggedly seek it. I would search for a love so deep it would be almost more than I could stand. In her book *A Natural History of Love*, Diane Ackerman describes the revered liminal space of desire between knights and ladies: "Only by staying wholly infatuated, damp with sublimated erotic passion, could one mine one's emotions inexhaustibly and strive higher, risk more, achieve nobler ends."[4] The wait is a game of perpetual arousal, explains Ackerman. Feeling convicted and holding onto a promise felt sexy in a culture that increasingly seemed stripped of the sacred.

Seeds of limerence planted in church went beyond hopeless romanticism because there was both hope *and* a sense of divine intervention. Everything could be a sign from God or the universe telling me this one guy was "the one."

Limerent love can even resemble a form of worship when the limerent object takes the place of God. Both the romance narrative and the Christian narrative suggest that if you find your one true love you'll live happily ever after, argues academic and romance novelist Catherine Roach in her book *Happily Ever After: The Romance Story in Popular Culture*. "The romance narrative is religious in its faith in the healing power of love, its focus on the beloved as 'divine' or of ultimate significance, and its mythic quest for love. 'Love is God' is the central dogma of such erotic faith," Roach writes.[5] The happily ever after is life everlasting for the believer in an idealized relationship with God. For me, it was winning the attraction of a beautiful man I'd put on a pedestal.

Purity Culture Feeds Romantic Longing

I was curious how and if purity culture (PC) had sparked limerence for other friends, so I reached out to the author of *Famished: On Food, Sex, and Growing Up as a Good Girl*, Anna Rollins, who grew up in a Southern Baptist church and attended a fundamentalist Christian school in West Virginia. She says both introduced purity culture in different ways. She signed a pledge in church and her parents encouraged her not to call boys or pursue them. "I would have these really intense crushes I would not pursue. I wouldn't stalk them because I was taught to be passive. But I would pray that God would turn their hearts. I think because I was taught I couldn't be an active agent in my life that contributed to some of my ruminations and fantasies of being saved. I was taught that men were like God, so in some ways, what I was looking for in romantic relationship was someone to save me—a type of Christ." When Anna was twenty-two, she married the first person she had dated seriously, and they lost their virginity to each other.

Purity culture perfectionism impacted her body image. "Even though we talked about God forgiving us for our sins, I don't think we actually believed in forgiveness. And if you don't believe in forgiveness, then there's so much pressure to be perfect all the time so that you're not thrown out of your tribe." For Anna, that developed into a complicated relationship with food and her body that resulted in several decades of disordered eating. To be a good woman, Anna was taught, she had to be very disciplined in her desires. When she applied that to hunger for food, that meant minimizing her appetite.[6]

Childhood friend and poet Jennifer Stewart says that from a young age she measured her Christian faith by her purity. As the daughter of my family's Baptist minister later turned Christian counselor, she grew up reading *Brio*, a Christian teen magazine her parents subscribed her to, attending an active youth group, and doing devotionals like *Lady in*

Waiting. When she was fourteen, her father took her to Chili's restaurant and gave her a key-shaped purity necklace rather than a ring (the "key to her heart") and a book that would shape her dating life for almost a decade, missionary Elisabeth Elliot's classic *Passion and Purity: Learning to Bring Your Love Life Under Christ's Control.* Its message: Battle your desires of the flesh and lay your longings on the altar before God. In the front of the book, her father explained how he hoped the book would be a guide for her romantic life.

In her anthologized essay "Girls with Big Boobs Can't Be Saints," Jen writes of this blueprint: "I had Elliot's book with which to wrestle my messy teenage longings into submission. I learned as the lingo said, 'to lay him on the altar.' To lay my own heart and each successive ill-fated crush from high school onward, on the altar and offer it up to God as a sacrifice because I could hear Elliot's voice in my head, reminding me of how much it pleased God to be a sacrifice."[7]

Jen and I moved away from each other at five years old, but our romantic lives were both affected by purity culture. "In my romantic nonlife, the type of man I was longing for were men who treated me in ways where there was no physical component to the attraction. That felt how a relationship that was 'Christian' should feel. It was the good spiritual person who's managed to disconnect their bodily impulses from this higher romantic thing," she told me.

During her early adult years, the longing never felt safe. "Everything about the Elisabeth Elliot model taught me that if you're longing for someone, you've made that person an idol, so you need to sacrifice that person."

For Jen, praying for that person she wanted to be with, perhaps her future husband, became a safe way of feeling connected to them, because in prayer she could both express feelings and keep them private. This spiritual practice created a sense of meaning when there was often none. "It feeds the feelings you want to feed," explains Jen, who lost her virginity to a Muslim at age twenty-four while serving as a missionary in Europe.[8]

Mary and I met in a Facebook limerence support group. She attended a purity ring ceremony in the nineties in Missouri at the Southern Baptist church where she attended youth group. Mary says for many years she prided herself on never dating or kissing anyone until the man she married (her current husband). Her best friends were younger guys and often the ones falling in love with her whose feelings she did not reciprocate. "I could have these close friendships and feel loved and adored and like I was still 'doing it right,'" she wrote.

She believes PC was fuel for a flicker of limerence that sparked when she was a child and that lasted into her current marriage. "I always had crushes on boys who were somehow beyond my reach, or so it seemed. The ones I could not breathe around, let alone talk to. Something made it easier to keep them on that pedestal. They were safe there. I developed this narrative that men must not really find me attractive because the ones I wanted did not want me back. And the ones who wanted me I didn't want back, so somehow they didn't count."

She attributes the link between PC and limerence to the belief of otherness between men and women. By segregating young women from men within faith circles, she says, we have othered one another in dehumanizing ways. This othering and the lack of intimacy that accompanies it fuel uncontainable longing.[9]

Josiah Hesse, fellow Colorado trail runner and author of the memoir *On Fire for God: Fear, Shame, and Poverty in the Christian Right*, grew up in rural northern Iowa attending a Pentecostal church, church camps, and many Christian music festivals. "There was so much ruminating on this fantasy human being that had been supernaturally chosen for you that you start to develop unrealistic expectations for who that person is going to be. I mean, inevitably, everyone who got married following that track was disappointed at some point because no one can live up to that standard. But it wasn't about that person, it wasn't about that relationship. It was about what was going on inside of your skull," said Josiah, who has also been diagnosed with ADHD.

He recalls repeatedly listening to DC Talk's song "That Kind of Girl" and Jars of Clay's song "Love Song for a Savior," and he remembers writing letters to his future wife thanking her for saving herself for marriage.

"We were taught again and again that virginity was a kind of currency. It was a transactional activity that you are giving someone as if you're giving someone a gift or an envelope of cash."

He recalls watching his pastor demonstrate this loss of value by chewing a piece of gum and then asking the group if anyone wanted it now that it had lost its flavor. "You've let God down. You've tainted that Holy Sacrament that he had set into motion before you were born," Josiah remembers the pastor saying.

Josiah fooled around with boys when he was in his teens, but he says, "I considered myself a virgin until I was like, nineteen, when I first actually had sex with a girl." There was a line to be crossed, he said, but no one knew exactly where that line was.[10]

Evangelical Christians aren't the only youth indoctrinated into longing. British novelist Salma El-Wardany, author of *These Impossible Things*, says her conservative Muslim community instilled a longing in her for an idealized partner. Salma was born to an Egyptian man she never knew and an Irish woman who converted to Islam and later remarried a Pakistani man. "My mother told me I could marry any man as long as he was Muslim. . . . I was constantly searching for this Egyptian heritage and this piece of me that was missing."[11]

Amy Chauhan says her religious upbringing in Sikhism influenced her to seek an ideal mate. "There was a deep desire to be purposeful about finding someone who would be good for my soul, which ended up being a tall order."[12] Amy lost her virginity at thirty-seven years old to the man she married after having a long-distance relationship with him for ten years.

Learning to Endure Long Distances and Not Settle for Second Best

My longing through high school was not sexual. I was mentally aroused by anticipation—the possibility of a dream coming true.

I didn't know what it felt like to sexually ache for someone. And, frankly, the idea of some guy thrusting his penis inside of me and then squirting his juice, as my grandma Velda called it, sounded absolutely repulsive. So, waiting until marriage to have sex didn't seem like a big deal—especially since I figured I'd be married shortly after college. If my peers thought it was an impossible goal, I would prove them wrong. I was the kind of straight-A kid who shot for the moon. By the time I'd graduated high school as salutatorian, I had twelve varsity letters in cross-country, swimming, and track. Endurance was my middle name. Sign me up for the longest distance. I would make it to the finish line even if I collapsed at the end.

During my freshman year in high school, I ran races with abandon. I didn't overthink anything, I just ran as fast as I could. Over the next couple years, as my body morphed so did my self-awareness. It distracted me. I had to dig deeper to run through the pain, to ignore the desire to stop. I wanted most to impress my father.

Suspicious I was holding back, my father told me that if I didn't collapse at the end of a high school cross-country race (3.1 miles) I hadn't tried hard enough. And so, I did—at most finish lines, I puked. I dropped to the ground. I passed out. It felt cathartic. Dutiful. Like an ascetic fast. My grandma stopped coming to watch me race "because it hurt too badly" to watch me finish.

I became very good at performing while disconnecting from my body, all in hopes of achieving that runner's high, a feeling of flow, like the awe felt after an orgasm. It's so rare, I've only felt the runner's high a total of three distinct times in my life.

Being a high achiever meant learning to ignore anxiety and hammer through physical discomfort. It was during those high school endurance races when I began to metamorphose into a version of the naked mole rat, which is impervious to certain kinds of pain and can survive without oxygen for more than eighteen minutes. The complete metamorphosis would take two decades of hookups, dozens of triathlons, seven marathons, and one Ironman to achieve.

But back then in high school, long-distance running training paralleled the "training" I received through purity culture. They both required me to suppress my physical desires through mental discipline. And the praise from male "coaches" for succeeding was the carrot I needed to keep going.

Delayed Gratification

To compound this pledge of celibacy, I had record amounts of willpower and a habit of saving. As a child, I saved my Easter and Halloween candy until the following season rolled around or until it was too hard to bite into. I would've made the children in the 1972 Stanford Marshmallow Experiment look impulsive. In that study, children were given a marshmallow and told that if they waited fifteen minutes without eating it, they would be rewarded with a second marshmallow. Researchers then tracked the lives of children who waited the longest for the reward of two marshmallows and found they tended to succeed more in academics.[13]

Were these children genetically programmed to delay gratification? A follow-up study in Rochester in 2012 corroborated the findings of the earlier one but also demonstrated how important environment is in willpower. Those children conditioned to feel they were in a reliable environment and could *trust* the researcher to deliver what was promised waited twice as long as those deemed to have strong willpower in the 1972 test.[14] I wanted that second marshmallow.

To me, the capacity to wait boils down to one word: faith. I was raised in a household where good things came to those who waited by parents who made good on their offers. If my parents couldn't keep their promises, they didn't make them. I would keep my promise too. And in the meantime, I would relish longing for the reward: an ideal match. A perfect match. The one.

Incomplete Tool Set

Despite a lot of disparaging press surrounding promise ring ceremonies, I felt empowered by mine—like I was in control of whom I would have sex with and when. I walked away from the experience believing my body was worthy of being treated with dignity and love. However, this message conflicted with the zeitgeist of my dating world when I entered college, which told me I didn't have to—and shouldn't—wait for love and a committed relationship to have sex. My mother's generation had fought hard so that my generation could enjoy abundant sexual freedom—to explore without inhibition. My mother's generation, but not my mother, had devoured *Sex and the Single Girl* by *Cosmo* editor Helen Gurley Brown, who declared, "If you're not having sex, you're finished."[15]

However, I would learn I wasn't as free as I thought. The tool set I wish I'd been given would've included the permission to sexually explore (sans alcohol) without shame. It would've centered women's pleasure as equally important as men's. It also would've defined consent as requiring a yes for permission to proceed. And, perhaps most importantly, it would've imparted the skills of listening to my body and respecting its pace and timeline.

Signing that purity pledge, and believing in it, was like agreeing to walk through quicksand and never sink. None of the church leaders anticipated or understood the secular college hookup culture I would enter in three years, where you couldn't play unless you paid and putting your drink down had dire consequences. They couldn't have anticipated the decline in church attendance of single twenty-something men in the early aughts. As my pool was shrinking, limerence became an even more secure place to hide.

CHAPTER 4

THE CHADS

May your mind inhabit your life with the sureness
with which your body inhabits the world.

—John O'Donohue, "For Longing,"

To Bless the Space Between Us

When *Sex and the City* first aired in June 1998, I was smack dab between my sophomore and junior years of college. In the first episode, Manhattanite columnist and socialite Carrie Bradshaw hooks up with an ex-boyfriend with whom she has no emotional attachment. She's sworn off looking for "Mr. Perfect." When the "self-centered, with-holding creep" offers her oral sex, she agrees, enjoys, and leaves before he's orgasmed. She tells the audience, "As I began to get dressed, I realized that I'd done it. I'd just had sex like a man. I left feeling powerful, potent, and incredibly alive. I felt like I owned this city. Nothing and no one could get in my way." This scene would galvanize an entire genera-tion, or two, of women to pursue sex like a man, to leave their feelings at the door and just fuck for fun and (feel obligated to) feel proud about it. After all, Charlotte, the only character in the TV show who reserves sex for commitment, is "punished" with an impotent man, Trey.

Over the next decade, detaching became an art, a talent women like myself tried to develop. Women's magazines published articles on how not to catch the feels.[1] One from *Elle* was titled "How to Have Casual Sex Without Getting Emotionally Attached, According to Science."[2] Entire conversations would develop in Reddit threads on how to emotionally disengage during sex with Chads, a slang term for stereotypical alpha males considered physically attractive, charismatic, and sexually successful.[3]

In freshman orientation August 1996 at my tiny but mighty liberal arts college of about one thousand students, we were all subjected to a discussion on safe sex. The magic word was *consent*—or simply the lack of "No!" It didn't matter if the sexual encounter was pleasurable or respectful as long as there was mutual consent.

One of our college's nurses taught us about dental dams (a weird-looking version of a female condom), passed out magnets with the campus police's information, and informed us of access to condoms in the health center. We were not warned about being roofied by college frat boys who often mixed our drinks at parties (practically the only social outlet on a heavily Greek campus).[4] I didn't learn about it until my college classmate ended up in the hospital the morning after getting drunk at a frat party and realized she'd been raped while passed out.

Nobody discussed how to handle the vulnerability hangover (on top of a real hangover) after the walk of shame: the snickering looks from peers on their way to breakfast as I slouched back to my dorm room still wearing my mini skirt, high heels, and red crop top the morning after hooking up with a boy in his room my senior year. Nobody acknowledged that disappointment and sadness were normal feelings to have after a hookup when the other person then pretended you didn't exist.

After months of feeling out of place among my freshman peers, who were getting drunk and hooking up on weekends, I wrote a letter to Dr. X, the psychologist I'd seen in high school while struggling with anxiety on the starting line at races. I explained the anxiety I had around kissing guys. I told him it sorta freaked me out to think of some guy in my face. In his reply, Dr. X wrote, "I don't think the 'phobia' you mentioned is necessarily unnatural or weird and happens to a lot of people. Feeling affection and love for someone is an internal process that involves so many things like your identity, your future and possible sexuality. Basically, if it doesn't feel right, it may not be right at this time. You are in control of your body." It was so affirming and freeing, unlike most feedback I'd received in high school or college, so I tucked it away in my keepsake folder of cards and letters that mattered.

The Rules of Hookup Culture

While my mother was reading *The Strong-Willed Child* to learn how to manage me, I wish she'd been preparing for my future by reading *Too Many Women? The Sex Ratio Question*, published five years after I was born.[5] The two authors were psychologists who had developed the Guttentag-Secord theory, which states that the sex in short supply (males or females) has greater power over the sex in surplus. This predicted my future dating pool, which Barbara Dafoe Whitehead described in her 2003 book (published a year after I graduated college) *Why There Are No Good Men Left: The Romantic Plight of the New Single Woman*.[6] In a low-sex-ratio society where women outnumber men, research shows men are more promiscuous and less willing to commit to a monogamous relationship.

The rise in the proportion of female students to males in college meant there were more women contending for limited male affection. Researchers noted that this increase in competition for a scarcer population resulted in women being more willing to lower their standards—which, in my case, often required a substantial amount of bourbon.

Sociologists Dr. Lisa Wade and Caroline Heldman in their 2010 article "Hook-Up Culture: Setting a New Research Agenda" wrote: "Some individual women may be capitulating to men's preferences for casual sexual encounters because, if they do not, someone else will."[7] This was never clearer to me than when my friend Sasha got in my face one Friday night, after several shots of Hot Damn! and vodka supplied by the frat boys, and declared, "He's going home with me tonight!" The "he" she spoke of was the same upperclassman with crystal-clear blue eyes and robust lips I had a crush on. She won (that night).

Hookups are really a game of status. "Hookup culture isn't about hooking up with someone you like. It's about hooking up with someone your friends are going to be impressed by," Lisa Wade, Tulane professor of sociology, told me in an interview.[8]

The sexual revolution never got around to valuing femininity, so hookup culture is just a male stereotype of what sexuality looks like, she told me. It's patriarchy in disguise, and it has excised all things we code as feminine. As the sexual liberation movement evolved alongside the sexual revolution, Wade explained, we conflated freedom with whatever men did—including sexual freedom. "When the daughters of the women who were young adults in the sixties and seventies got to college in the mid-1990s, they applied that logic—women's liberation is the right to do anything men do. You apply that to sexuality and you get hookup culture," Wade said.

In her research of US college hookup culture for her book *American Hookup*, Wade identified several governing rules, namely, that both parties consider the hookup meaningless.[9] "You can flirt and be friendly before a hookup, but during a hookup sex should be hot but not warm. Extended eye contact, caressing, and slow kissing is off script in hookup culture. Sex is supposed to be great but not sweet.... After a hookup, no matter how friendly you were before, you're supposed to take a step back from how friendly you are—produce some aloofness with that partner to make sure nobody is confused about what happened: It was just sex and it wasn't anything more than that."

The ambiguity combined with the lack of accountability fostered by hookup culture created the perfect recipe for limerence fueled by hope and uncertainty. The first time I recall a boy dry humping me happened to also be the occasion of my first college kiss. I was twenty years old, a sophomore, studying abroad in Strasbourg, France, with other college classmates. I'd drunk half a bottle of cheap merlot at the soccer players' apartment party. The soccer players were notoriously hot (and often high), and I had never yet been invited to one of their parties.

It was two in the morning and I lay clothed on the cold tile floor in the kitchen as the brown-eyed junior with a firm ass and thighs that could squeeze a lemon humped me while his housemates were passed out in their rooms. I started laughing as he began to moan, surprised at how easily he got off. "Stop laughing," he berated me. But I couldn't. I wasn't physically aroused. I felt embarrassed, ashamed, and amused all at once. Of course, I didn't dare admit any of that to him. I told myself it should feel like I'd earned a badge to have hooked up with and been desired by such a desirable male.

But the morning after my first overnight hookup, I didn't feel that way either. I woke up early while he was still snoring and hopped the train back to the home stay where I lived with a French family and my best guy friend (I'll call him Mon Ami), a lanky, curly-haired classmate with Clark Kent glasses and a nearly perfect French accent. I ugly cried on his bed as I tried to expunge myself of shame by sharing with him all the lurid details. He comforted my hungover self with an embrace (I'd later long for from the other side of the world) all while verbally cringing and saying he really didn't want to hear anymore.

Why did feeling desired by one of the most popular jocks on campus also feel trashy? For the rest of our semester abroad, the hot soccer player would make fun of me in front of his friends or hang with his ex-girlfriend when we weren't drunk and hooking up. He called me Phil McCracken. In class one day, I found a photocopied picture of his middle finger (recognizable by the ring he wore) in my backpack. I convinced myself that he was teasing me like I'd been told boys did in junior high when they liked you. For the first time in my very limited history of sexual experiences, I felt both successful and disposable.

But it all went against the messages I'd been fed. If I could compete and play just as hard as any man, why did I feel so awful?

The "Alpha Female"

Although I'd been conditioned through church to believe in a divine plan, sitting patiently for it to unfold went against the other doctrine my parents had instilled in me: If it's to be, it's up to me.

When I moped after placing last in a swim competition, my mom sat me down and firmly explained, "We are a family of ass kickers, so go out and kick some ass." Things that accrued real meaning were those things I actively sought—even if that meant imaginative plans that went no further than my head.

By the nineties (my high school and college years), Title IX had finally taken root in universities across the country, the pill was readily available in college clinics, women were outnumbering men in college, and the term *girl power* was coined. Fem-punk bands like Riot Grrrls and Spice Girls elevated the phrase.[10] Cultural propaganda told me I had the sexual freedom to sleep with whoever and remain independent. In "None of Your Business," Salt-N-Pepa sang: "If I wanna take a guy home with me tonight, it's none of your business."

I was born on the cusp of the "alpha girl" era—a generation of women clinical psychologist Dan Kindlon researched and wrote about in *Alpha Girls: Understanding the New American Girl and How She Is Changing the World* (2006).[11] This was a generation of girls who (and whose parents) weren't afraid to put themselves in positions where they could get knocked down because they were confident enough to rebound.

But as girls were evolving, becoming more flexible and more comfortable in roles and experiences previously reserved for boys, boys and their roles and experiences—and expectations—remained largely static. This reality is precisely why hookup culture worked as it did and perhaps why bitter incel (involuntarily celibate) communities began developing in the late nineties.[12] As more and more women began to exercise greater freedom in their sexual expression, more and more men felt entitled to sex. The sexual revolution was backfiring.

The girl power that rose up in the nineties represents, according to Kindlon, "emancipated confidence."[13] It worked well in the classroom, on the sports field, and in climbing the corporate ladder. But it didn't teach women how to deal with their natural inclination to bond with the hot soccer player they'd confidently just hooked up with who now wanted nothing more to do with them.

Sociologist and psychotherapist Dr. Leslie Bell, author of *Hard to Get: Twenty-Something Women and the Paradox of Sexual Freedom*, noticed this dissonance among her college female students and clients in the early aughts. "I was hearing a lot more confusion than clarity. Young women were feeling they weren't meeting those sort of new ideals, new frameworks, the kind of woman they 'should be.' One of those frameworks was a sense that she should feel very comfortable with her sexuality, to understand her desires and be able to act on them," she told me.[14]

Exchanging and Masking Desires

Girl power failed in the dating world dominated by hookup culture, where both men and women were forced to cripple their emotions (often with the help of alcohol) to avoid being seen as clingy.

In the nineties, the National Institute on Alcohol Abuse and Alcoholism (NIAAA) noted college binge drinking was on the rise, particularly among women. For the average-sized woman, that meant four drinks or more in two hours, and for the average-sized guy, five drinks.[15] My own college experience with alcohol reflected this trend. Alcohol gave me superpowers to overcome the high school yearbook superlative I was voted: "Most Naive." Before college, I'd never had more than a sip of my grandma Nancy's Bloody Mary and the shot of peppermint schnapps my mother offered me before prom. "This is for your date!" she said tersely, as if softening my bitchy attitude would make my shy date's night more enjoyable.

With a few drinks in me, I could cross boundaries with a crush that my sober self wouldn't touch. Although my college was (then) in a dry county, we never ran out of alcohol. Nobody wanted to drive to a liquor store at ten o'clock on a Friday night, so "alcohol runs" meant stocking up on Boone's Farm Strawberry Fields and Jim Beam (manufactured just down the road) ahead of the weekend.

"I never swallow" took on a variety of meanings in college. While my college cross-country teammates were restricting their food intake, I was developing sexually restrictive habits. It was my way of maintaining an even playing field. Desire, hunger, discomfort—I became adept at silencing all those voices. It would take me twenty years before I'd notice the damaging effects of this cognitive dissonance, this suppressing of my authentic voice, but in college, I began seeing it eating away at my friends in the form of anorexia and bulimia—some had mild cases and others required hospitalization. It was a form of control (dare I say, self-punishment) when women felt out of control while ironically attempting to feel empowered through sexual agency.

One cross-country teammate began starving herself to counter the sexual feelings she was acting on with her high school boyfriend (to whom she lost her virginity). She told me she punished herself for fulfilling (giving in to) one desire by restricting another: hunger. "I self-identified as the 'good girl' and believed that's how I was pegged in my social circle. I felt that identity was slipping away. Controlling what I ate was what I clung to in response to something else I wasn't controlling—my desire to have sex. I felt guilty that it felt so good," she told me.

Throughout college, I received rose-scented letters from Grandma Velda. One contained a wallet-sized card with my name in bold type across the top followed by its supposed translation, "Worthy of Love," and then the Bible verse Joshua 1:9, "Be strong and of a good courage; Be not afraid, neither be thou dismayed: for the Lord thy God is with thee whithersoever thou goest" (KJV). Alpha females may have been assertive and persistent in the classroom, on the athletic field, and at the frat parties, but I'm not sure we really believed we were worthy of love.

And so, because I didn't believe it, my pattern of dissing quiet nice guys in high school continued in college. My dad, also a quiet nice guy, got tired of hearing me bemoan how nice these men were and watching me reject them. One summer evening when I was in my twenties, my high school friend Bob picked me up as his date for his friend's wedding, and my dad did what he'd never done before: Offer the guy advice. "Treat her like shit!" he called from the family room while we stood in the doorway. Bob looked at me perplexed. "I'll explain later," I said.

Rather than grapple with my own emerging sexual desires in a college culture where ambiguous drunken hookups ruled and nice guys seemed boring, I often chose to fall into more limerent traps by longing for some elusive goal.

In "Ode on a Grecian Urn," nineteenth-century poet John Keats writes, "Heard melodies are sweet but those unheard are sweeter."[16] I pinned this poem to the bulletin board in my dorm room and unconsciously embraced the idea that anticipation for what we hope to come is more appealing than the thing itself. I never imagined I'd become the middle-aged romantic flutist frozen in motion on the Grecian urn, "a burning forehead, and a parching tongue."

I feasted on passionate stories of longing that often ended tragically: Tristan and Iseult, Pip and Estella, Marcel Proust and Albertine, and, of course, Romeo and Juliet. They taught me that suffering, something I intimately knew from endurance running, was a prerequisite for passion.

CHAPTER 5

ANCHOR MEN

*I never knew until that moment how bad it could hurt
to lose something you never really had.*

—Kevin, in *The Wonder Years*

Many of us attach anchor memories that shape our self-image and future romantic pursuits to key romantic interests we had in our early lives. Psychologists call these self-defining memories. Often, the individuals linked to these memories arrived in our life at major transition times: graduation, death, relocation. The following three Anchor Men, as I like to call them, resulted in three particularly painful back-to-back-to-back rejections that left me feeling stuck.

Anchor Man 1: Mon Ami

Mon Ami was the Peter Parker, Clark Kent, Bruce Wayne in my story. But when people asked, as they did frequently, why we weren't more than just friends, I'd shrug and say he was like my brother. Mon Ami felt too emotionally close and familiar to be physically attractive to me. He knew I'd fart if I ate too much delicious camembert and that I was a bitch if I didn't get out for a run each day. He knew I was afraid of the dark and that I hated when he pursed his lips pretending to be French.

For spring break our sophomore year studying abroad, we traveled throughout France together aboard train after train, just the two of us. We visited the Louvre in Paris, rented bikes in Pontorson and rode to Mont-Saint-Michel, toured the castles Chenonceau and Blois in the Loire Valley, and hung out (clothed) on the Riviera's nude beaches in Saint-Raphaël and Nice.

One evening in Nice felt almost like we were on a date. In a children's clothing boutique, I bought a stork-printed peach dress for the infant daughter I envisioned. To dinner, I wore a long pink cotton dress and the fleur d'oranger (meant for cooking) I'd bought that afternoon. On the menu of the tiny nook of a restaurant we chose named La Closerie was the most orgasmic appetizer: *chèvre chaud à la lavande avec miel*. We splurged on a room at a chain hotel, La Mercure (much nicer than the dingy hostels we'd stayed at), and slept together in the same bed for the first time. I'm not sure whether my awful sleep that night was because of my heightened awareness of Mon Ami's body next to mine or the sound of the waves crashing on the beach outside our window.

Following our semester abroad together, our junior year came and went, and our friendship remained steady. But by winter of our senior year, after a fall semester competing and training together on the cross-country team, our friendship was simmering with tension, even though we had never been physical in any way. Mon Ami was leaving for France again for a monthlong internship, and the potential of a romantic relationship between us felt like it was looming—as was my last semester of college.

"Un des aspects le plus merveilleux du francais, c'est que le mot 'ami' est ambigu-exactement comme notre rapport," Mon Ami wrote in a card at Christmas our senior year, 1999. Translated: "One of the most marvelous aspects of French is that the word 'friend' is ambiguous, exactly like our relationship."

My anxiety about my future was the most intense I'd ever felt, and it was manifesting through hairpulling (trichotillomania). I began seeing a therapist on campus, and my doctor prescribed Paxil for my anxiety (fifteen years later I would be diagnosed with ADHD). I was applying for English as a second language (ESL) teaching and running-coach positions all over the world. This potential relationship with Mon Ami felt as ambiguous as my future. I felt a sense of a chapter closing and I was panicking about doing all the things right.

On my birthday, a few days before Valentine's Day, the buildup of four years of walks and talks and confusion culminated in the stairwell of his apartment with Bruce Springsteen's "Dancing in the Dark" blaring on the stereo from the kitchen, where our friends were partying. Mon Ami removed his glasses, pulled me against his lean body, stooped down in his Chuck Taylors, and kissed me for the first time.

During that last semester of college, our relationship resembled a dahlia flower blooming: Every time it expanded, it contracted a little bit. He was hot and then cold, then lukewarm and then cool. There were no dates, just a handful of sober hookups at his place or mine, all amid our decisions about the future. I went further with him sexually than I had with anyone else because I trusted him. And through that exploration together, I felt connected and dependent on him and vulnerable in ways new to me.

But his behavior was confusing. At graduation, he invited me to join him on his family's beach vacation—just a month after he'd said we shouldn't see each other anymore. I was perplexed. But I vacationed with him at the beach anyway.

On our last night, he kissed me while we lay on the beach in the soft, pearly Gulf sand under the moonlight. The rhythm of the waves matched the undulations I felt slowly filling my body with warm hope for our future. A few days later in the airport, he would kiss my tear-damp face goodbye, and I would feel anxiety's familiar grip in my throat. I didn't want to let go, and something in my gut knew that he had never held on to begin with. For the first time, I felt like I was in love with someone who loved me back. But he was leaving for a research position on a French island, and I was moving to Indiana for a graduate assistant cross-country and track coaching position.

On August 25, 2000, two weeks after the family trip, he wrote me: "Although we meet many interesting people in our lives, only a few really influence us, change the course we take (or would have taken), and I certainly count you among these people in my life. I too don't know where we'll end up, but I speak from experience when I say that, in my opinion, the best policy is not to focus on the past or even the future, but just to relish the bond we share right now. That is, I think, the only way to make it last."

I felt such contradiction in his words. He sounded like he wanted our bond to last, and yet, was he referring to our friendship or our romantic relationship?

In his letter he reflected on a story we'd read in French class. "Do you remember that passage from *Swann's Way* when Proust describes how awkward we feel in new bedrooms until habit silences the clock? I kind of feel that way, except I haven't even found the room I want to move into yet."

For Proust, as it does for limerents, love doesn't exist in real time but only in anticipated or remembered time. And so, I sought to preserve our bond. On my dresser, I set up a shrine: a card from Mon Ami, an Eiffel Tower ornament, a photo Mon Ami's sister took of us embracing on the beach, a seashell from our trip, the bottle of fleur d'oranger, the green and yellow beaded necklace he made for me. I listened on repeat to CDs of artists he'd introduced me to: Mary Chapin Carpenter and Belle & Sebastian. It was a way of praising the relationship I so badly wanted to continue cultivating. That fall we talked a few times on the phone. I sent him letters. There was no Skype and email wasn't that popular yet. For Christmas, he sent me a giant atlas book. An invitation to visit, I thought. And two weeks later, after a phone call where I sensed his distance and he likely sensed a subtle panic in my voice, the letter arrived from the other side of the world:

> *My reason tells me that being with you is a once in a lifetime opportunity, but my heart tells me that I'm not truly in love. . . .*
> *With lots and lots of affection,*
> *Love, . . .*

Through tears, I called my parents and read the letter to them. I called Mallory and Lynn, who were now engaged, and read it again. I read it over and over on my own. I dissected every word and tried to decipher the few words he'd scribbled out with pen.

For most people, that letter would have been enough to nail the coffin shut. But, instead, I focused on all the things he didn't say: "I never want to see you again." "I don't love you."

When all indications suggest hope is lost, limerents facing unrequited love continue to grasp for hope. In the great feminist writer Simone de Beauvoir's book *The Second Sex,* she recalls a friend trying to make sense of the long silence of a distant lover: "'When one wants to break off, one writes to announce the break'; then, having finally received a quite unambiguous letter: 'When one really wants to break off, one doesn't write.'"[1] I could relate. It didn't matter whether Mon Ami had written or not, I'd find a way to convince myself it wasn't over.

Neurological Yearning

For several decades, psychologists have been arguing that romantic love is less a feeling and more a drive, like thirst, thus harder to control. Romantic love emanates from the parts of our brain in the mesolimbic reward system, buried deep below the part of our brain that makes rational decisions. Dopamine, the neurotransmitter that lights up pathways in the reward systems of the brain for people on cocaine and opioids, also lights up the same pathways for people experiencing romantic love—even years after rejection.

Following Mon Ami's letter, there was no follow-up phone call or letter on either side. That was it. I was furious and heartbroken. I felt left without recourse. I felt all those feelings of grief Elisabeth Kübler-Ross described in her landmark 1969 book, *On Death and Dying*: denial, anger, bargaining, depression.[2] Everything in my neurological system wanted to seek him out and mend the gap.

We are prewired to long for lovers, even the ones who have broken our hearts. In a 2010 study, researchers found that when heartbroken individuals were shown photos of their rejecting beloved interspersed with photos of other familiar individuals, their brains lit up upon seeing their rejecter in the same places others' brains did when exhibiting romantic passion. Photos of the rejecters also stimulated a part of the brain that encouraged the rejected to obsessively evaluate gains and losses.[3]

"There's some part of the brain that says, 'Your partner is really rewarding.' You get extra dopamine when you try to reunite with them," Dr. Zoe Donaldson, neuroscientist and professor at the University of Colorado Boulder, told me. I visited her lab and watched her students place wires into the brains of prairie voles, fuzzy little rodents who are monogamous (a rarity in the animal kingdom). They've found that the vole's brain starts releasing dopamine when the creature presses a lever (signifying a decision has been made) requesting access to its partner. When the vole anticipates the reward of being with its mate, it gets dopamine.[4]

This is similar to what neuroscientists say is happening in the brain of someone experiencing limerence: Anticipating a response from an LO, fantasizing about being with that LO, or scheming ways of (re)gaining the LO's attention provides a hit of dopamine.

In other words, my hyperfixating on Mon Ami was a simple fact of my animal nature. Like the voles, I would not give up hope. I rationalized how with time—after he'd spent time in a different "bedroom"—he'd return to me. After all, even my professor had told me he thought we'd get married. Call it magical thinking or mindlessness.

Anchor Man 2: The Artist

Within a year of that goodbye letter, I became involved with an older man who was arguably more traditionally Hollywood attractive than Mon Ami if less academically successful. But the Artist was equally ambiguous in his communication style and elusive. He was a brilliant abstract landscape painter moonlighting as an insurance salesman. And, damn, could he sell.

The first time my mom saw a photo of him, she said he looked like Superman. After that, I could never look at him any differently. His brown eyes were darker and sharper than Mon Ami's and his clean-cut hair was almost black. This former college football player, with squared shoulders, a dominant brow ridge, and a jawline that rivaled Gregory Peck's, was thirty, seven years older than me. The soft-spoken Artist was my coworker's brother, whom I met the spring following Mon Ami's letter. He would become my most potent LO and the attraction would last for almost eighteen years. He became to me what Mr. Big was to Carrie in *Sex and the City*: an unwinnable object I fantasized about winning.

That following Christmas break, I dared myself to ask his brother for the Artist's number so I could call and ask him out to dinner. Some people jump off bridges and wonder if they'll land on their feet. I called men who I considered completely out of my league and asked them out (this wasn't the first time, but he was certainly the best looking). Both my mother and I almost peed our pants when he said yes. My self-esteem soared. I felt electrified when I was around him, sometimes I felt so nervous I was speechless (and gassy).

A few weeks after my first dinner date with the Artist, I stood at my grandfather's hospital bedside as he died. During the many hours I'd spent with Gramps fishing, we'd talked about Maya Angelou's poetry, the difference between trolling and casting, the art of cooking good bacon, love and death. He was a poet disguised as a dentist. On one early-morning Michigan fishing trip, he told me he wanted a bagpiper at his funeral. He was the first person close to me to die. I counted the seconds between his rattling breaths until his lungs filled with fluid and there was no more room for air. Then, Gramps was gone.

Stunned, I reported it to the nurse and called my dad. Grandma Nancy wailed beside me, "I'm going to be so lonely!"

Something about my grandfather falling ill in late December and then dying in January coincided with my budding relationship with the Artist that my brain could not shake loose. It was almost as if being with the Artist would help me recoup a loss or make things even. The Artist and I saw each other whenever I was home in Cincinnati. That equated to about one visit a month for about three months. Then in April 2002, the introverted Adonis who smelled like clean laundry went as my date to Mallory's wedding. After the wedding, while I lounged in my yellow chiffon bridesmaid dress on his couch and listened to Miles Davis's album *Kind of Blue*, he kissed me for the first time—the kind of kiss that melts you from the inside out. It felt like he sucked all the air out of me. Like a drug addict chasing the most mind-blowing hit, I would seek to repeat that moment for almost two decades.

Shortly after coaching was done that season, I moved back to Cincinnati, and our relationship grew deeper. For another three months, we spent time picnicking in parks, hiking, dining out with friends, making out while watching movies. I spent the night at his apartment at least once a week. He respected my boundaries and moved slowly. He knew I was reserving sex for a committed relationship. He also knew I was leaving at the end of the summer for a teaching job in Grenoble, France. One morning, when he had to leave early for work, he kissed me goodbye while he thought I was still asleep. For years, I would tell myself that kiss meant he loved me.

A week before I left, we picnicked in Eden Park. I asked all the questions. "What about us? Do you want to be exclusive while I'm gone? Will you come visit me?" I felt like I was dangling again in yet another ambiguous relationship that I desperately wanted to materialize.

"Of course, I want to see you again," he responded. "But let's see how this year unfolds."

The next eight months unfolded with me being the only one calling and sending cards and packages. He responded to my emails (sometimes after weeks went by) and answered my phone calls (when he wasn't working).

My emails became pleading. "So, has work finally swallowed you whole? Did you get my very lengthy email? I told myself you were working on a painting to express your thoughts rather than writing me."

My God, I sounded desperate!

What he wrote in his last email to me were the kind of crumbs that I would subsist on for years: "I guess we will have to see what happens when you get back here. I am definitely not opposed to seeing you when you come back at all. It would be quite nice, actually:)"

And he *would* see me, but not for another six years.

Even though I was returning home from France, uprooting from a community I'd strived so hard to develop left an odd sense of homesickness, and the Artist's silence made my homecoming feel even emptier and directionless.[5]

I would later learn how big transitions trigger old attachment wounds, which activate sharp bouts of limerence. When there is something about our current situation that reminds our system of the original separation or loss we felt, and we encounter someone who has a familiar "energetic signature" as that period of loss, the protective part of us screams, "Attach to him or die!" Our survival physiology creates the perfect chemistry—a cocktail of dopamine and vasopressin, a hormone (released to counter stress) that promotes feelings of trust, love, and loyalty—to convince us of an attachment that exists only in our head. Something about the Artist withdrawing reminded me of my grandfather's death.

Muddled Grief

The New York Times Magazine essayist and my friend Lauren DePino has written extensively about the intersection between heartbreak and grief.[6] The man she thought she was going to marry dumped her the day after her grandma's funeral. "I was catatonic. I needed him to come back for my survival—or so that's what I believed at the time. Later, I'd understand that it was my grandmother I was grieving, and that I was projecting it all on him." Her grandma had been like a mother figure to her throughout her life.

"When I felt him pulling away, I let parts of myself die in an attempt to keep him. I created this fantasy that he would come back." She even argued with the psychics who said he wasn't coming back. "I wouldn't accept his goodbye. I saw him, at the time, as my salvation," she said.

"I thought that true romantic love could shield me from loss because it was eternal. It was all muddled with spiritual love," she told me. DePino grew up going to Catholic music camp and singing at funerals. "I had a nun tell me God was calling me to be a nun. I thought about saying yes, as God was the only partner who wouldn't die or leave you." She eventually became a music minister. "I was very familiar with helping others deal with grief but terrified of experiencing it myself," she said.[7]

The National Institutes of Health defines loss as a state of deprivation from a motivationally significant person, place, or object.[8] The definition of what the Artist was to me.

Anchor Man 3: The Soldier

My ultimate fairy tale began developing the summer I returned from France. As for Cinderella and Dorothy, for me, it involved a woman trying on a pair of shoes. She had come into the Cincinnati running-shoe store where I worked looking for a pair of comfortable walking shoes. We struck up a conversation that led to her telling me all about her son, a West Point graduate stationed in Baghdad. She showed me a picture of him, a blue-eyed blond in Dress Blues, and then proceeded to give me his address, which she had conveniently typed on little slips of paper to hand out to people like me—people who might send an encouraging letter to her son.

In August 2003, he and I began a year of correspondence by letter that fueled my limerent fantasy about a mysterious soldier. About twice a month, a letter from Baghdad would arrive at my new home in Boulder, Colorado, where I'd moved for a teaching job and to pursue my athletic dreams. My soldier often wrote his letters on the back of yellowed papers printed with Arabic writing and a silhouette of Saddam Hussein's face. The Soldier's penmanship was impeccable and he signed off, "Yours in Christ." We discussed poetry, music, career aspirations, God, and family. He described the bombs he'd narrowly escaped and how many rounds of ammunition and wired-together mortar rounds he'd recovered from homes his unit was instructed to raid. I shared tales of my blunders made during my first semester teaching ESL at the university and while attending massage therapy school.

"Where do you like to be kissed?" I asked in one letter.

"In the rain," he wrote back.

By winter 2003, our correspondence moved from letters to emails to phone calls. The first time I heard his voice after many months of correspondence, it breathed a calm, gentlemanly voice into his articulate written responses to my often-prying questions. A full year after we started writing, he was granted a few months' leave. He decided to travel around Europe and asked me to meet him there—anywhere.

This is it, I thought. My soldier. My savior. My most romantic pen pal. I'd waited, and he had arrived. He may not have found my glass or ruby slippers, but his mother's shoe purchase had helped me land my fairy-tale guy at last.

I hesitated at first to fly across the world for a weekend to meet a man I had only ever seen two pictures of. My father, the practical, nonromantic type, surprised me: "You can use my Delta airline miles. Go. Meg Ryan would do it, wouldn't she?"

I suggested to the Soldier we meet in Paris. We set a date: Labor Day weekend. He suggested we meet in a confessional booth in Notre-Dame. I had other ideas. I sent him a CD titled *Saint-Germain-des-Prés* and an excerpt from Hemingway's *A Moveable Feast*. He would know it was me: I would be sitting in Café de Flore reading the book.

After sitting on pins and needles for thirty minutes in the corner of the café sipping a glass of Sancerre, a gentleman who looked vaguely like the one in the photos sauntered in and sat down next to me. He hugged me. I could barely look at him those first ten minutes. Like the time my dad shaved off the mustache he'd had for fifteen years, it felt like an out-of-body experience associating a very familiar voice with an unfamiliar face.

He got a Coke. (It was always Coke or hot chocolate. He didn't drink alcohol. And he always prayed before his meals.)

About halfway through dinner our first night in Paris, a grin grew on the Soldier's face. My back was to the open window. "It's raining," he said. A few hours later, he kissed me on the Pont des Arts overlooking the Eiffel Tower. We returned to our many shades of pink hotel room in the Latin Quarter that looked out on Rue Saint-Sulpice.

The long weekend exceeded my romantic expectations. We became "that couple" kissing on Paris park benches I had only photographed on previous trips to Paris and mentally photoshopped myself into. There was listening to jazz sitting in red velvet seats in tiny, smoky bars, picnicking on the lawn beneath the Eiffel Tower, exploring the ancient meandering streets hand in hand (him always chivalrously walking on the outside closest to the traffic), and late nights discovering each other's curves and rhythms. It was the romantic scenario I'd envisioned to lose my virginity, but I still had my guard up with the Soldier.

One afternoon as we strolled through the Tuileries Garden and watched the children float their brightly colored boats and old ladies walk their little dogs dressed in plaid vests, the soft-spoken Soldier asked the question, "What will become of us?" He was headed back to the States for about a year before he'd have to deploy again.

I said that I wanted to continue a relationship back in the States but to wait till we were both home to start, not live out a fantasy in Paris. "And you?" I prompted.

"I have never found anyone like you and don't ever want to again," he responded.

My heart leapt with excitement and my body collapsed at the same time. I suddenly felt like what I'd wanted for so long stood in front of me, yet something about me withdrew from his open arms, care, and attentiveness. It was so unfamiliar, it all irked me. Limerence had faded. My mind kept wondering, "What is he hiding?" In reality, I was the one hiding from accepting love.

Our long-distance relationship developed into weekends at bed-and-breakfasts in the romance breeding grounds of Santa Fe, New York City, and Aspen. Our relationship flourished, nourished by the symphony at Carnegie Hall, gifts of Victoria Secret lingerie, passionate airport kisses (one up against a wall in the Albuquerque airport women's restroom), and the crackle and scent of pinyon pine campfires. By January 2005, we'd both said "I love you" to each other—him first in a letter.

Before the Soldier, I'd never uttered those three words to a man other than my father, brother, and grandfather. I meant them when I said them. The Soldier was patient, genuine, wise, and generous—something I'd never been attracted to. He now signed his letters, "Entirely yours" and "Absolutely yours."

He adored me and showed it in every way. And I didn't know how to absorb it because, frankly, I didn't think I deserved it.

For days after our Valentine's Day weekend in Santa Fe, I could still feel and smell his damp cold cheek pressing into mine after he'd ridden several hundred miles on his motorcycle to meet me in Santa Fe, a convenient meeting point equidistant from Boulder and his military base in Texas. That visit, he asked me, "What would you say if we got engaged?" My stomach flipped and my throat tightened. Panic poured into my gut like stiffening cement, crushing all my butterflies. He had both feet in and I had one foot out.

"Don't ask hypothetical questions," I said flippantly. And he never did again.

I thought I was in love with him, but the perfectionist in me kept fixating on his flaws that irritated me: the time he rearranged my magnetic poetry on the fridge to be in alphabetical order, the time he shushed me in the symphony, the way he'd knock his West Point ring on a table, the time he pushed away our family dog when she was seeking attention. The fact that he was balding in his mid-twenties (I know, so vain). These shouldn't have been deal-breakers, but they grated on me. The truth was, I didn't know how to receive love now that I had love and commitment, so it was easier to poke holes in the fabric of attachment between us.

My mom called with advice. "You can keep dating and searching until it's a marry now or never situation, or you can 'settle' with someone and make the best of it."

Her advice echoed in my brain. Mallory had just had her first child, a daughter. I thought about the peach dress I'd bought for my own little girl. I began to worry I was messing up a once-in-a-lifetime opportunity with the Soldier.

Nine months after the Soldier's return to the States, he was deployed again, this time to Kuwait. It was July 2005. We planned to spend our last weekend together before deployment in Virginia where he was stationed. By the time I got there, I could sense that he had already begun to mentally deploy; all the while, I was hopelessly engaged in trying to connect. With imminent separation looming, my longing had kicked in full throttle.

After much deliberation and angst, including many miles on the running trails talking it out with a friend, I had decided I was ready to have sex with him that weekend—for him to be my first. Maybe I asked him if he wanted to have sex. Maybe I told him I was ready to have sex. I don't remember what I said precisely, but I do remember the Soldier saying, "No." How deeply embarrassed I felt by the stark rejection. Like I'd shown up naked to the wrong party. Now that I had both feet in, he had one foot out.

Maybe he didn't really want to. Maybe he didn't think I really wanted to. Maybe he wanted to leave this time with no strings attached. Maybe he was simply being respectful because he didn't know what he could promise once deployment was over. I felt a sense of panic—like knowing something you loved was beginning to unravel and you wouldn't be able to repair it because someone had run away with the string. I flipped over and quietly cried myself to sleep.

He kept his valuables and a few copies of *The Economist* in a large chest. By the end of that weekend, it was clear I was not part of that chest anymore. Staring out the window on the airplane home, I anxiously cried, feeling like I had left something behind—even if it wasn't my virginity. But I would wait for him. And maybe he would decide when he got back from war that I did belong in that chest of his.

University politics on the subject of campus rape state that consent means a verbal yes. It's no longer the no that is given much attention. In my case, the Soldier's no caused more scar tissue than any running trail fall I'd ever endured.

Never would I have thought that that no would put me on the track I found myself for almost fifteen years—avoiding attentive and secure loving relationships where there is potential to say yes. I had come so close to living out the fairy tale I'd imagined, to having the Superman I believed existed, to finally having sex in the safe and loving relationship I desired, and yet it ultimately all unraveled that night my offer to have sex was rejected.

Halfway through his deployment, the Soldier returned to the States for a two-week leave. We met in our usual haunt, Santa Fe, but jumping in bed with him that first night felt like jumping in bed with a stranger. The Soldier made it clear that he had plans for his future, and he wasn't 100 percent sure I was still part of them. "If it's in God's will, it'll happen," he said.

The uncertainty was crushing. After that brief but honest weekend, it would be another six months before we'd see each other again. But by that point, neither of us had either of our feet in. Friendship is what he offered when we met for ice cream at Christmas in Cincinnati, but then I never saw him again.

Self-Defining Memories

My unique experiences with these three men left me with what psychologists call self-defining memories. Connecticut College psychologist Jefferson Singer dedicated his life to studying these important integrated memories. He found they are defined by five elements. They are vivid, emotionally charged, repeatedly recalled, linked to other memories, and focused on lasting goals or unresolved conflicts.[9] "Certain memories keep their emotional power because they are linked to goals and desires that are still most important in our lives," Singer writes in his book *Memories That Matter: How to Use Self-Defining Memories to Understand and Change Your Life.*[10]

Although I couldn't see it at the time, the Soldier's rejection scarred me deeply.

But I would find new ways to manage my fear of uncertainty, abandonment, and disempowerment, just as Grandma Velda had learned to manage hers after watching her fifty-four-year-old husband die of a heart attack in bed. While she threw herself into a clinical depression, I would throw myself into the arms of hot alpha males, where I felt wanted, even if for only a night. In a dating world where the one rule that dominated was to have lots of meaningless consensual sex, I would create my own rules. My target audience: mysterious emotionally unavailable avoidant types, often charming narcissists.

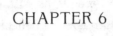

CHAPTER 6

PETER PANS

Pan described to Wendy, "You know that place between sleep and awake, that place where you still remember dreaming? That's where I'll always love you. That's where I'll be waiting."

"Just always be waiting for me, and then some night you will hear me crowing."

—James Barrie, *Peter Pan*

For about a decade following the Soldier's rejection, I went on dates with about fifty men. I got a euphoric high from my ability to attract noncommittal Peter Pans (fully knowing they likely wouldn't materialize into the ideal relationship I sought), fool around with them, and still maintain my virginity. Falling for Peter Pans—the charismatic yet highly insecure, adventurous, reluctant-to-commit, often vulnerable narcissistic types—was a fabulous escape from the real, vulnerable intimacy I'd tried and struck out on.[1] I wasn't afraid to be left again if I kept my virginity. Some screwed-up equation in my competitive head made me feel like I was winning. But I was the only one keeping score.

I was flexing that longing muscle: strengthening that part of my brain that enjoyed fantasizing about Peter Pans who had already fled and future options I had only yet stalked on Match.com and other social media platforms.

Boulder was home to an abundant supply of potential limerent objects. And there was always a steady stream of visiting pro athletes. The city was a magnet for Peter Pans with chiseled abs whose resting heart rate and VO$_2$ max numbers rivaled Lance Armstrong's. Usually, their number of college degrees exceeded their number of committed relationships.

Back then, men outnumbered women in Boulder. They dated seasonally: a mountain biker chick in the fall, a backcountry skier in the winter, a trail runner in the spring, a whitewater kayaker in the summer. If you didn't match their activity, they didn't have time for you, so they'd move on and likely not explain why. They were in no rush to settle down. Boulderites seem to think they are permanently young.

Empowerment

After striking up a conversation at a December triathlete-dominated holiday party, Stefan and I exchanged a series of friendly text messages that led to a meeting for coffee turned invite to his hotel room at the historic Boulderado to "watch TV" because it was "too cold" for him to venture out three blocks to the café I'd proposed. It had become a tug-of-war, and I was game. Instead of the café, I suggested we meet in the hotel bar for a beer—more appropriate, I convinced myself, than going straight to his room.

I was already perched at the bar drinking a Vesper cocktail when he sauntered in, seeming inconvenienced by the commute down a flight of stairs. He wore tight black jeans and a blue silk shirt. "You want to see my wallpaper? It's this beautiful floral print," he asked me in a thick foreign accent. Really, I thought, that's all you've got? We bumbled over silly small talk about triathlons, watts, racing, his training schedule, and why he was visiting Boulder: "Want to see my bike fit measurements? The detail is incredible," he said.

That sounded like a good enough excuse to go up to his room. I followed him up the same steps Helen Keller had climbed. I followed him into his room but left the door cracked in case I needed to yell for help.

He could read me. We spoke different native tongues, but fear is universal.

"What am I going to do?" he asked. "Rape you? My reputation would be ruined."

He acknowledged the risk and so I took it. After twenty minutes of making out, I admired his completely nude sculpture, elongated and aroused on the bed as I stood topless beside it. Practically every inch of his finely tuned and toned body was void of hair. "You didn't finish your job," he chided me with a smirk.

"I think you can finish it," I said. "You *are* an Ironman World Champion." I replaced my bra and top and walked out feeling incredibly empowered. And just like that, I'd lived a confident Carrie Bradshaw moment, but I felt only marginally fulfilled—was he the pawn or was I?

I was drawn to these attractive, highly ambitious alpha males who, I knew full well, expected me to have sexual intercourse with them. But it was never about sex for me. It was about control in the form of a challenging escape. It was a game I loved to play with Peter Pan players— unwinnable objects. Men with narcissistic traits and an avoidant attachment style were crack to my limerent self: I was flattered by their initial interest in the form of inconsistent love bombing and hint dropping, intrigued by the challenge of them pulling away once they'd sucked me dry for their narcissist supply, and relieved knowing they were never going to give me the true emotional connection I deeply feared.

Limerents feed a narcissist's hunger for validation and worship. But once their fragile ego is filled up, the limerent is forgotten, seen as intolerable, or relegated to backup status for when the narcissist needs a hit.

With an ever-increasing number of people with narcissistic traits reportedly in the dating pool, the question begs to be answered: Are narcissists creating more limerents or are limerents creating more narcissists?[2]

I felt empowered when I hooked up with men I barely knew and came out the other side seemingly "unscathed" (or so I thought), with my virginity (as I defined it—no penile penetration) still intact.

Hookups also gave me fodder for limerent fantasies. I would go home after a hookup, research the hell out of the guy, and develop an entire storyline about how I might win his affection. The research also helped me assuage the guilt I felt for being so physically intimate with someone whose tattoos I knew but whose values I didn't. Occasionally, a Peter Pan would inspire a poem that I would write and send him. When I was bored or stressed at work, I would drop into reverie, thinking about a single brush of his hand against my ankle. Sometimes, like many who lean on limerence for mood regulation, that's even how I fell asleep at night.

While friends like Mallory and Lynn were getting married and having kids in our late twenties, I played the role of their single friend from whom they sought out adventurous dating stories. Unlike them, I could keep hopping from one LO to another (in limerence terms, this is called "transference"). All the while, I was unknowingly creating an unhealthy pattern of dissociation during intimacy (a seed that had been planted in college)—training my body to become desensitized and emotionally detached while still being very physically sexual. These situationships were like the intervals I'd run in training sessions to build my tolerance to the pain of the marathon that is dating in a sea of Peter Pans.

I was overcome with the fear of missing out and making the wrong decision, so I continued to serial date. This looked like: (A trail run followed by a beer) × 3 + (A booty call) + (Silence). Studies show that immediately after finishing a race, ultrarunners have significantly higher levels of oxytocin, the cuddle hormone released after childbirth and orgasm, in their blood than they did at the start.[3] There was something about putting myself through discomfort for several hours, I guessed, that made me want to bond.

Strengthening a Neural Pathway

For a decade, a steady stream of situationships kept me just satiated enough to not change my patterns but hungry enough to keep chasing. I collected experiences with fascinating men. I dated two men who shared my birthday (one the same day and year), a Trader Joe's grocery clerk who took me flyfishing, a philosophy professor who taught me about opera, a waste management baron, a bayou-born alligator-wrestling policeman who liked kink, a retired CIA spy, a veterinarian whose dog humped my leg, and enough engineers to start a firm. I hooked up with Russian, Singaporean, Brazilian, French-Senegalese, Polish, Peruvian, Czech, Canadian, Chilean, and Indian men. A grandson of a senator, a man who wrestled an escaped convict to the ground, a grandson of a Communist revolutionary, and a mountaineer who'd traded in guiding elites like the vice president to securing transactions at a local strip club. I dated men ten years younger and fifteen years older and a Matthew, Mark, and John. I made out with men in a friend's closet at a Christmas party, at lakes, in parks, inside tents, on a boat on the Thames, at a secluded beach in the Virgin Islands, in a one-room cabin, in a running-shoe store stockroom, and on too many dance floors to count.

I had *a lot* of fun, and I remain friends with some of these guys I met on my decade-long dating spree collecting experiences.

But all the while, I continued strengthening the neurological pattern of chasing the feeling of early romantic love I'd established as a tween: the spike in dopamine followed by a depletion of serotonin (the same neurochemical loss found in obsessive-compulsive disorder). There was also an increase in nerve growth factor, which strengthens synaptic connections—a boon to my old pal limerence, who loved to create associations between disparate clues to keep hope of the LO's interest alive.[4] I was bingeing on falling in love. The more often I associated anxiety with excitement and excitement with love, the stronger became the neural pathways that led me away from a safe, enduring relationship.

I related to "The Darling," the main character in Anton Chekhov's short story, who finds her identity in her devotion to a series of love objects whose talents she'd inflated. "She was always fond of someone, and could not exist without loving," wrote Chekhov.[5]

Guys who were transparent, who were kind or complimentary, I continued to flee like the plague. *His hands are too rough. His weekends are too open to plans with me. He can't keep up with me on a trail run. His kitchen sink is too full of dirty dishes.* It was almost like I went searching for their flaws while somehow overlooking the enormous red flags the Peter Pans were waving. Instead, my limerence goggles had me running toward them mistaking the red flags for a festival. I found some perverse sense of security in involving myself with noncommittal men whose ambiguous silence was softly signaling rejection.

At the same time, I pushed away men who were giving, like the Soldier. I didn't mind giving or receiving from friends, but I didn't like feeling the unspoken obligation like when you owe someone for a "favor." It felt wrong to be pursued, like I was not working hard enough or investing in the challenge—or lack thereof. I felt safer longing to receive love.

Some people enjoy the feeling of liking (anchored in the present), and others enjoy the feeling of wanting (anchored in the future or the past). Although these feelings are encoded slightly differently in the brain, they both trigger dopamine release. My brain bathed in wanting, like a pig in mud.

Psychiatrist Ethel Spector Person, in her book *Dreams of Love and Fateful Encounters*, described my romantic pursuits. Some lovers, she wrote, "prefer the chase to the quarry. Excitement is everything, realization nothing; they may become love addicts, whose lives are parsed out in rapid alternations of erotic excitement and disappointment."[6] I would later learn that *love addiction* was an actual term psychologists used to help people with this self-destructive conquest behavior, this desire to "win" the beloved. The overlap between love addiction and limerence is remarkable.

What Is So Seductive About Limerence?

In November 2023, *Cosmopolitan* ran a feature that described limerence as "a self-regenerating obsession that rarely leads to a healthy relationship." Embedded in the article was a poll asking readers how they felt about "falling in limerence." Eighty-seven percent picked the answer "Give me an all-consuming romantic infatuation or don't waste my time."[7]

But why are so many women like me motivated to pursue something so torturous that has been clinically proven to generate anxiety and depression and lower self-esteem?

Investigation into the motivations for pursuing unrequited love sounds like complicated physics problems. For example, approach–avoidant gradients, established by researchers Paul Wong and Susan Pfeiffer, measure "the extent to which intimacy with the beloved and potential rejection is at a distance, approach tendencies should maximally exceed avoidant tendencies." In other words, the less likely you feel you are to face rejection, the more likely you are to pursue (even mentally) a relationship with an LO. Sounds a lot like what other psychologists refer to as the Cyrano situation, named after Cyrano de Bergerac's infatuation with Roxanne, where the blissful hope of a romance developing balances out the risk of rejection. Roy Baumeister and Sara Wotman call this "falling upward," which totally seems fitting for limerence, where you place your LO on a pedestal.[8]

Clues

It's easy to overestimate the probability of an LO's reciprocation if you're like Sherlock Holmes's assistant, routinely combing the world for positive clues to keep your hope alive: a wink, an encouraging word, a text reply. The seeker often has a confirmation bias and interprets any ambivalence as positive while ignoring any negative signs.

A psychologist who studies mind wandering, Dr. Giulia Poerio told me she wonders if there's something unique about the brains of people who fall into limerence that causes them to interpret facial expressions differently from how most people do.[9] For example, when I saw a face in a crowd that remotely resembled the Artist's (with his sharp dark eyes in narrow ovals, high cheek bones, and chiseled jawline), my heart would skip a beat. Scientists think it's a resurgence of the oxytocin I felt when I emotionally bonded with him that causes his facial features to be burned into my brain and my brain to always be subconsciously scanning the crowd for him.[10]

For those wired for limerence, our LOs have a signature "glimmer" that acts as a supernormal stimulus, a romance accelerant, a sensory cue to which our response is exaggerated.[11] In nature, animals that react to supernormal stimuli include birds, which will neglect their own eggs to obsessively brood a porcelain egg, and large beetles, which will attempt to copulate with beer bottles decorated with glass beads. I had become the bird trying to hatch the porcelain egg.

In her book *Love and Limerence*, Dorothy Tennov describes how keenly aware a person experiencing limerence is of an LO's body language, particularly their eye gaze.[12] Psychologists call the tragedy that results from misreading cues a "Giselle situation," based on the ballet *Giselle*. In Act One, the peasant girl Giselle "misinterprets" cues of affection from an engaged nobleman named Albrecht, who deceives her in his disguise as a peasant. One scene depicts Giselle plucking petals from a daisy. In French (the supposed origin of the game) this is called *en effeuillant la marguerite*, and there are five choices: "He loves me a little—a lot—passionately—madly—not at all." Ultimately, Giselle falls madly in love with Albrecht, goes insane, and dies of heartbreak. In Act Two, Giselle is summoned from her grave by the resentful Wilis, the ghosts of unmarried women who died on their wedding nights after being betrayed by their lovers. The Wilis take revenge in the night by dancing men to death. When Albrecht delivers flowers to Giselle's grave, Giselle saves her beloved by holding off the Wilis until dawn. Giselle's selfless act exonerates her from becoming one of the Wilis and forces Albrecht to live with the burden of his deception.[13]

Damn Albrecht for deceiving Giselle. One of my closest high school friends Lilly fell in love with a man she met on Tinder who professed to be someone he wasn't. She invited the supposed "Special Forces" guy